You will find:

- *A free subscription to our e-newsletter,* Smart Publications Update

- *The latest facts and findings on natural hormone replacement*

- *A complete catalog of all our health enhancement books*

- *A directory of healthcare practitioners knowledgeable in alternative medicine*

- *Many other articles you may find of great interest and value*

SMART PUBLICATIONS™
Your Source For Alternatives

NATURAL HORMONE REPLACEMENT

FOR WOMEN OVER 45

– by –

Jonathan V. Wright, M.D.

& John Morgenthaler

SMART PUBLICATIONS™
POST OFFICE BOX 4667
PETALUMA, CALIFORNIA 94955

707/763-3944 (FAX)
www.smart-publications.com

Natural Hormone Replacement

For Women Over 45

by Jonathan V. Wright, M.D. and John Morgenthaler

Published by:
Smart Publications™
PO Box 4667
Petaluma, CA 94955

fax: 707 763 3944
www.smart-publications.com

Library of Congress Catalog Card Number: 97-65916
First Printing 1997
Printed in the United States of America
Second Edition

Library of Congress Cataloging in Publication Data
Natural Hormone Replacement For Women Over 45
Jonathan V. Wright, M.D. & John Morgenthaler
Includes Index & References
1. Menopause Treatment
2. Hormone Replacement
3. Health
4. Aging
Preassigned LCCN: 97-65916
QP251.W26 1997 613.9'5 93-22227

ISBN: 0-9627418-0-9 $9.95   Softcover

Warning - Disclaimer

Smart Publications has designed this book to provide information in regard to the subject matter covered. It is sold with the understanding that the publisher and the author(s) are not liable for the misconception or misuse of the information provided. Every effort has been made to make this book as complete and as accurate as possible. The purpose of this book is to educate. The author(s) and Smart Publications shall have neither liability nor responsibility to any person or entity with respect to any loss, damage, or injury caused or alleged to be caused directly or indirectly by the information contained in this book. The information presented herein is in no way intended as a substitute for medical counseling.

. . . .

ACKNOWLEDGEMENTS

I'm very appreciative to:

John Morgenthaler
*without whom this book might not have been
published for another few years.*

Lane Lenard, PhD
*for his remarkable ability
to read enormous numbers of research papers
and reorganize them in a highly understandable way.*

Maureen Williams, ND, & Trina Seligman, ND
extraordinary scholars, physicians, and library sleuths.

Alan Gaby, MD, Professor at Bastyr University
*superbly accomplished practitioner of natural medicine,
and my long-time partner in teaching seminars for health care
practitioners, for his review and discussion.*

Devaki Lindsey Berkson, DC
(twice Chiropractor of the Year in California)
for her review of key portions of this book.

Holly (my wife)
*for her incredible patience and support
while I worked on this book.*

—Jonathan V. Wright, MD
TAHOMA CLINIC, KENT, WASHINGTON 1997

ACKNOWLEDGEMENTS

... and special thanks to:

Jonathan Wright, MD
*the source of inspiration for this book, whose clarity
of thought is greatly appreciated and admired.*

Lane Lenard, PhD
for his talent and hard work.

Ward Dean, MD
*my partner in many publishing projects before,
for introducing me to Jonathan and for his dedication
to the causes instead of his ego.*

Will Block
for adjusting my sights on a much bigger picture.

Holly Hamm
for her patience, love, and intelligence.

Doug Casey
for making ERIS happen.

—John Morgenthaler
PETALUMA, CALIFORNIA 1997

About The Authors

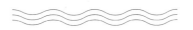

Dr. Jonathan Wright is the best-selling author of *Dr. Wright's Guide to Healing With Nutrition* and *Dr. Wright's Book of Nutritional Therapy* (600,000 copies sold.) He is medical director of the Tahoma Clinic in Kent, Washington and has treated over 2,000 women with natural hormone replacement since 1982. Dr. Wright has also been a monthly medical columnist for *Prevention* (1976-1986) and *Let's Live* (1986-1996) magazines. Along with Dr. Gaby, Dr. Wright has taught *Nutritional Therapy in Medical Practice,* a four-day intensive seminar for health care practitioners, annually since 1982. This course is based on the Wright/Gaby research library, a compilation of over 35,000 medical journal articles dating from 1920 to the present.

■ ■ ■

John Morgenthaler is the co-author of *Smart Drugs & Nutrients* and *Smart Drugs II: The Next Generation* (together 150,000 copies sold internationally.) He is also co-author of *Better Sex Through Chemistry* and *STOP The FDA: Save Your Health Freedom*. John has appeared on the *Today Show, Larry King Live, 20/20,* and *Phil Donahue,* and has been interviewed in *Time, Newsweek, Playboy, Washington Post, USA Today, New York Times, Los Angeles Times, San Francisco Chronicle, The Economist, Rolling Stone, Mademoiselle,* and many others.

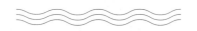

*"By studying the organic patterns of heaven
and earth a fool can become a sage.
So by watching the times and seasons of natural
phenomena we can become true philosophers."*

LI CHU'UAN
YIN FU CHING

— *(Approximately 735 A.D.)* —

∎

AS QUOTED BY JOSEPH NEEDHAM IN
SCIENCE AND CIVILIZATION IN CHINA,
VOLUME 5, CAMBRIDGE UNIVERSITY PRESS, 1983

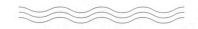

TABLE *of* CONTENTS

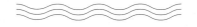

P R O L O G U E

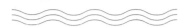

JOAN DAVIS WAS WORRIED about growing older. "It's not my age; I'm actually enjoying being 51," she said. "The children are grown; I have more time to myself and to be with John. I'm enjoying my grandchildren, and I've started painting again. I hadn't done that since my first daughter was born. It's not even these wrinkles, though I wouldn't mind a few less."

"What really bothers me," she said, "is the thought of not being able to take care of myself when I'm 99 ... I do plan to be 99, you know. So, I've decided to consider hormone replacement therapy, and I almost decided to go with the standard treatment when my sister ... Linda Salzburg, you know her ... told me about the natural hormone replacement she just got here. It sounded so right, so here I am."

"How did natural hormone replacement 'sound right' to you?" I asked.

"Well ... you know, Linda had been on Premarin® and Provera® before she came here. She said it just didn't feel quite right, but she couldn't put her finger on why. Many of my friends say the same thing. So, when I heard about replacing my hormones with exactly identical hormones—instead of those horse hormones—I thought, 'What a concept!' Makes 100% good sense. Besides, why use anything that increases the risk of cancer?"

"Your periods have stopped?"

"Oh yes, two years ago. I didn't have nearly the problem Linda had—non-stop flashes, depression, all that—I just had a few hot flashes, a little irritability and sleep trouble. I went to the natural food store, added some extra vitamin E, calcium-magnesium, and lots of herbs for menopause—and that was it, no problems since."

"No hormones of any kind?"

"No. I've been keeping up on health matters for years, ever since our children were small, and I read too many things about the added risk of cancer from 'estrogen' replacement. My doctor told me that using a 'progestin,' too, cuts down that excess risk, but that sounded too much like 'hitting yourself with a hammer and taking aspirin to stop the pain,' if you know what I mean."

"So, what changed your mind?"

"Time—and maybe age and observation. Now that our youngest is gone—she actually left when I was going through menopause—I've had more time to read and look around outside our immediate family, and it's made me more and more uneasy. A dear aunt is starting to lose her memory. The doctors say maybe it's senility, maybe Alzheimer's; it's too soon to tell. My mother's well, but, you know, she's just not as strong and energetic as I want to be when I'm 74. And so many of my friends' mothers have had heart problems, cataracts, macular degeneration, hip fractures, strokes, cancer ... and it's not just their mothers, but their older sisters, too. Like I said, I've been doing everything I can to stay healthy for years—so I decided to reconsider hormone replacement."

"Hormone replacement's only part of a 'staying-as-well-as-we-can-while-getting-older' program," I started.

"Good grief, I know that! I may not have been here before—we just moved to Seattle last year—but I've read your articles since the 1970s, and your books, and lots of other health books, too. To save time, I'll tell you what I'm doing already."

"Thank you."

"I cleaned up my diet—and my family's, too, when they'll pay attention—years ago. We have as much fresh, whole food, as I can find, hardly any from packages and cans. I make as much as possible from fresh materials. When we buy anything with a label, I trained the kids to screen out anything with food colors, flavors, preservatives—though they're not doing so well now that they've left home—except for my oldest. She reformed the minute she found out she was pregnant with her first. Now where was I?"

"No food chemicals."

"Oh, yes. We don't have any sugar or artificial sweeteners in the house, or in anything we eat. We eat lots of vegetables and fruits, though it certainly took a long time to convince John. Of course, only whole grains. We have fish regularly, some beef, but more chicken and turkey. I've started looking at soy products, but it's sometimes hard to find them without preservatives."

"There are more good ones in natural food stores all the time. Please keep looking. Soy seems to help prevent many diseases, cancer, for example."

"That's what I've read. Let's see, we have raw nuts and seeds for snacks: walnuts, sunflower seeds, almonds, and so on. I use only olive oil for cooking, and I've had John install a water filtration system in every house we've been in to eliminate the chlorine and as many other pollutants and additives as possible. Now, here's my list of supplements ...."

She gave me an extensive list that included a high-quality multiple vitamin-mineral, extra calcium and magnesium, vitamins C and E, ginseng, ginkgo, and several other items.

"You haven't missed a thing," I said. "Your diet and supplements should help you prevent quite a bit of health trouble. What about exercise?"

"Except when the children were very small, I've always walked regularly or played tennis."

"About the only things missing from your prevention program are natural replacement hormones," I observed. "With everything you're doing already, are you sure you want to take them?"

"I considered bolstering my supplement program further instead, adding more of that *anti-aging* stuff," she answered. "I'll probably do that anyway, but I read about estrogen replacement preventing senility, and that did it for me. I want the best chance I can get of going out with all my marbles."

"That's been really exciting research the last few years," I said. "First in animals, now people. There's every reason to expect it'll be the case for men, too, with appropriate hormones, of course ... but back to you. As you know, hormone replacement has been known to help prevent heart and artery disease and osteoporosis for women for some time. Now, researchers are finding a mental

13

health connection, too. But what would you predict if you knew that there are *hormone receptors* on nearly every cell in our bodies, not just on heart, artery, bone, and brain cells?"

"Hormone receptors—those are places that hormones activate?"

"Yes."

"And they're on nearly every cell we have?"

I nodded. She thought for at least a minute, and then asked, "Are you trying to tell me that hormone replacement will affect every cell, every organ we have: skin, blood, lungs—everything, and help it all stay younger, or at least slow down the aging process everywhere?"

"Seems logical, doesn't it? And if we use *natural* hormone replacement, with hormone molecules that are identical in every way to what our own bodies make, in the same proportions and following the same timing, we're much less likely to cause problems."

"I hadn't thought of it that way. Hormone replacement therapy is *whole-body therapy,* not just bone or heart treatment."

"Exactly."

She frowned and thought again for a few seconds. "There's no long-term experience or research at all on natural hormone replacement, though, is there?"

"No and yes. No, these hormones have not been 'tested' in the large, expensive, double-blind studies that some modern scientists can't live without. But, there's 30 to 40 years experience using patentable 'hormone' replacements—Premarin,® Provera,® things like that—and there's very little doubt that natural hormone replacement can do much better than those mismatched molecules."

"And the *yes* part?"

"Natural hormones have been thoroughly checked out for tens of thousands of generations of women. Nature seems to have settled on them as the safest possible."

"Can't argue with that."

"Of course, the other alternative is no hormone replacement at all."

"More heart disease, osteoporosis, senility, and who knows

what else! No, I've made up my mind, give me the prescriptions, please."

"Did Linda tell you that natural hormone replacement isn't just natural estrogens and progesterone, but DHEA and sometimes testosterone, too? And that there's testing involved to make sure all the hormones replaced aren't too high or too low?"

"But just right for me. Sounds like Goldilocks and the three hormones," she said.

"Sort of. Even natural hormones need to be monitored. Too little won't help, and too much is more likely to give you unwanted symptoms."

"I understand. Some of this is a little complicated. I wish there were more information, a book I could read about it all. Is there one?"

"Not yet." I wrote the prescriptions and marked the lab forms.

"I'll just ask questions every time I'm back—which won't be too often, though, because I'm planning to stay well!"

• • •

Like Joan Davis, you're planning to stay healthy, too—or you probably wouldn't be taking the time to read this book. In the chapters that follow, you'll find all the information Joan and others have asked about over the 15 years I've been working with natural hormone replacement (NHR) therapy to help women stay healthy, both before and after menopause. I hope it answers your questions (and maybe your doctor's, too), and helps you to stay well for both your own sake that of your family.

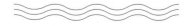

C H A P T E R 1

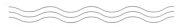

Welcome to the Age of
Natural Hormone Replacement

FROM THE TIME SHE first enters puberty until the end of her last menstrual period, every woman is keenly aware of the constant hormonal changes going on inside her body. Except during the months of pregnancy, she will experience the complex interplay of the estrogens,[1] progesterone, and other hormones, ebbing and flowing on a usually regular 26- to 28-day cycle, until she reaches her late 40s or early 50s.

The menopause, "the change," or "the M-word," marks the end of the cycling of these hormones. While current medical practice often treats menopause as an age-related disease, like high blood pressure, women know it's really a natural and inevitable transition from one stage of life to another. Puberty marked the beginning of reproductive life, and menopause marks the end of it.

In 27 years of medical practice, I've worked with hundreds of women making this transition. Each woman deals with the changes in her body and her life in her own way, with reactions ranging from joy and fulfillment ("It's finally over!"), to resignation and acceptance, depression ("I'm not young any more"), discomfort, and chronic illness. There is no "typical" reaction pattern.

"Menopause" is defined as beginning after a woman's last period, but her familiar monthly pattern of hormone secretions actually starts to change years earlier, usually as she reaches her early to mid-40s. The years before periods stop forever are called perimenopause. Like a rapidly spinning top that wobbles as it slows,

---

1. Human estrogen is actually composed of three hormones: estrone, estradiol and estriol.

the hormones of the menstrual cycle go out of balance during the perimenopausal years. The hormonal "wobbling" becomes ever more erratic with the years, and by the time most women reach about age 51 to 55, the "menstrual top" has stopped spinning altogether.

Although it's usually shorter, the perimenopausal phase can last as long as ten years. During this time, some periods may be heavier than others. Cycle length may start to vary in women who've been perfectly regular for years. Cycles without ovulation occur more often, and some periods of bleeding are completely missed. Skipping twelve periods in a row "officially" confirms the milestone labeled "menopause" for most women.

CHANGES OF MENOPAUSE

• Depression
• Disturbed Sleep
• Poor Concentration/Memory Lapses
• Heart Disease/Atherosclerosis
• Thinning Skin
• Hot Flashes
• Osteoporosis
• Irregular Menstruation
• Vaginal Thinning/Dryness
• Painful Intercourse
• Slow Healing
• Reduced Libido

Irregular menstruation is only one sign that menopause is imminent—and often not the most disturbing one. Because estrogens and progesterone have profound effects throughout women's bodies, perimenopause is often marked by a wide variety of well-known and usually unpleasant symptoms, reflecting the body's response to its changing hormone balance. These include hot flushes (or "hot flashes"), night sweats, insomnia, a general dryness and thinning of the vaginal area, noticeable aging of the skin, diminished sex drive, anxiety, forgetfulness, depression, and other mood changes.

As the years after menopause go by, the risk of serious cardiovascular disease (high blood pressure, heart attack, and stroke) rises dramatically. Cardiovascular disease is far and away the leading cause of death in postmenopausal women, dwarfing all other causes, including cancer. Osteoporosis risk also increases after menopause. Thinning of bones leaves many older women vulnerable to fractured hips, wrists, spine, and other bones.

For some, "creeping forgetfulness" is an unwanted accompaniment of the years after menopause. For a few, loss of memory and "thinking power" gets so bad that self-care becomes difficult or impossible. New but increasing amounts of research have linked some of these losses to the relative absence of estrogens, progesterone, and other menstrual cycle hormones.

The Age of Hormone Replacement

None of this is pleasant, so it's no surprise that women are usually quite eager to alleviate unwanted symptoms and reduce the long-term risks associated with the menopause. Our generation seems particularly eager to find a medical solution to menopausal woes. Certainly symptoms and suffering aren't any worse than those experienced by our mothers and grandmothers, but there has been a change in attitude.

Members of the "baby-boom" generation have learned to expect medical solutions to "problems" like menopause. Growing up with birth control pills, our generation is the first in human history with the option of spending the entire fertile lifespan taking hormones to control reproductive function. Why should post-reproductive, "menopausal" life be any different?

Indeed, why should it? The major medical solution to menopause for more than three decades has been a variation of birth control pill technology known (somewhat inaccurately) as "estrogen" replacement therapy, or ERT. The logic behind ERT is quite simple. If a lack of estrogen is causing body systems to malfunction and making life generally miserable, why not just replace the missing estrogen?

The promise—and apparent simplicity—of ERT is attractive: a life free from hot flashes, vaginal pain, and other discomforts of the perimenopause. And, after menopause, ERT seems to offer crucial protection against at least two major causes of death and disability in older women: cardiovascular disease and osteoporosis. So attractive is this promise that one form of "estrogen"[2]

2. Premarin isn't exactly the same as human estrogen, which is why the "estrogen" in ERT is in quotation marks. This is an extremely important point that will come up often.

replacement, Premarin,® has been among the most frequently prescribed drugs every year since the early 1970s. In 1996, more than 22 million prescriptions were written for Premarin® in the United States (about twice as many as those for such popular drugs as Prozac® and Zantac®), which was worth nearly $370 million to its manufacturer, Wyeth-Ayerst Pharmaceuticals.

For the most part, ERT's promise has been fulfilled. Although scientific evidence is conflicting, most women who have taken supplemental "estrogen" (either as Premarin® or other types) have reported they feel better. Their doctors have told them their risk of heart disease and osteoporosis is lessened. However, conventional ERT can cause unwanted effects for some women, including withdrawal bleeding, fluid retention, bloating, headache, nausea, anxiety and irritability, vaginal discharge, and even allergy to ERT itself.

A Disturbing Undercurrent

Despite the overwhelming clinical and marketing success of Premarin® and other forms of synthetic "estrogen," there has been, almost from the start, a disturbing undercurrent of doubt about the safety of conventional "estrogen" replacement therapy. That doubt can be summed up in one word: *cancer.*

The first cancer associated with "estrogen" replacement therapy was cancer of the endometrium (the lining of the uterus). If we look up Premarin's® legally required labeling,[3] the first thing striking the eye is a large boxed-in area strategically placed to make sure it's the first thing we see when we read this document. The actual wording of the Premarin® cancer warning is shown in the box on the next page. A variation of this warning appears on the

3. You can find a drug's labeling on a small sheet of paper that comes packaged with every drug. If your pharmacist does not automatically give you a package insert, or PI, when you fill a prescription, you should ask him/her for it. The PI, which usually comes folded like a miniature road map and is printed in annoyingly tiny type, contains lots of interesting information about a drug. For example, it includes everything the drug company would like doctors to know about their drug that the FDA will allow them to say. It may also contain a few things they would rather not say that the FDA insists that they do. You can find PIs for most drugs in a book called the *Physicians' Desk Reference,* or *PDR,* which you can purchase or find in any library.

··

Official Premarin® Warning Label

Estrogens Have Been Reported to Increase the Risk of Endometrial Carcinoma

Three independent, case-controlled studies have reported an increased risk of endometrial cancer in post-menopausal women exposed to exogenous estrogens for more than one year. The risk was independent of the other known risk factors for endometrial cancer. Therse studies are further supported by the finding that incidence rates of endometrial cancer have increased sharply sincce 1969 in eight different areas of the United States with population-based cancer-reporting systems, an increase which may be related to the rapidly expanding use of estrogens during the last decade.

The three case-controlled studies reported that the risk of endometrial cancer in estrogen users was about 4.5 to 13.9 times greater than in nonusers. The risk appears to depend on both duration of treatments and on estrogen dose. In view of these findings, when estrogens are used for the treatment of menopausal symptoms, the lowest dose that will control symptoms should be utilized and medication should be discontinued as soon as possible. When prolonged treatment is medically indicated, the patient should be reassessed, on at least a semi-annual basis, to determine the need for continued therapy. Although the evidence must be considered preliminary, one study suggests that cyclic administration of low doses of estrogen may carry less risk than continuous administration. It therefore appears prudent to utilize such a regimen.

Close clinical surveillance of all women taking estrogens is important. In all cases of undiagnosed persistent or recurring abnormal vaginal bleeding, adequate diagnostic measures should be undertaken to rule out malignancy.

There is no evidence at present that "natural" estrogens are more or less hazardous than "synthetic" estrogens at equi-estrogenic doses.

---

labels of all "estrogens" not occurring naturally in humans, as well as the popular estrogen "patch."

There are Two Key Points in this Warning:

First, taking Premarin® for more than a year increases the risk of cancer of the endometrium by as much as 14%. Well-controlled studies have shown that the risk of endometrial cancer is cumulative, rising at a rate of four to five cases per 1,000 Premarin® users with each year of use. By the fifth year of Premarin® use, a woman might be facing a 2% risk, and by her tenth year, her risk might be as high as 4% or 5%. Second, other forms of "synthetic" estrogen carry about the same risk.

After many years of prescribing "unopposed estrogen" ("estrogen" with no other accompanying hormones), and probably causing tens of thousands of women to develop cancer as a result, physicians finally discovered that the risk of developing endometrial cancer due to estrogen replacement can be reduced by also replacing missing progesterone. Progesterone can block or "oppose" estrogen's cancer-causing tendencies.

Nature and Creation* have known this all along! (Sometimes, we in medical practice are a bit slow). As long as there have been human bodies, and very likely longer, estrogen and progesterone have participated in the intricate dance of the menstrual cycle. The rise and fall of each is intimately linked to the rise and fall of the other. They're like two sides of a coin. To replace one without the other is an invitation to trouble which was too long ignored by nearly all medical doctors.

The "progestogen" (NOT progesterone, but more about that later also) physicians most often prescribe now is also a synthetic one called medroxyprogesterone, which goes by the brand name Provera.® The combination of synthetic "estrogen" and Provera,® called "hormone" replacement therapy, or HRT, is standard practice among most doctors today.

While the addition of Provera® may minimize the risk of endometrial cancer due to patentable "estrogen," it does nothing to lessen another serious risk of "estrogen" replacement: breast cancer. Women on a regimen of standard HRT using synthetic "hormones" like Premarin® and Provera® may increase their risk of breast cancer by as much as 30%, according to some estimates. In real numbers, this means that for every 1,000 women using one of these drugs, 300 will eventually develop breast cancer from the HRT itself.

Not good odds, but many doctors observe that without "estrogen," the risks of heart disease and osteoporosis, and their complications, are far greater.

---

* One author, John Morgenthaler, would prefer to say, "Nature worked this out a long time ago."

The Natural Hormone Option

While there may be truth in this observation, it ignores what should be obvious. Natural estrogen and natural progesterone provide all the benefits of the synthetic forms—and more—with many fewer side effects, while increasing your risk of endometrial or breast cancer very little, if at all!

If you've not heard much about natural estrogens and progesterone, you're not alone. It's not likely your doctor has either. Because natural hormones cannot be patented for the same reasons you can't patent natural air, water, or vitamins, there's little or no incentive for the pharmaceutical industry to spend the $200 million (or more) necessary to patent, develop, and test even one of these hormones, and then get it approved by the Food and Drug Administration (FDA). Many more millions would then be necessary to bring an approved hormone to market, and then promote it to doctors and their patients!

A patent grants an exclusive right to sell the patented product for 17 years. Unpatentable natural hormones can be manufactured and sold by anyone, as long as standards of purity and consistency of dose are met. Have you noticed any Wyeth-Ayerst brand Vitamin C or Bristol-Meyers-Squibb brand melatonin on drug store shelves? No? I'm sure you know why: it's far more profitable for these huge companies to develop patentable variations of vitamins, hormones, and other naturally occurring metabolites, even if they don't work nearly as well (and cause more trouble than) the original natural molecule.

Many doctors—who have little enough time to keep up with the world of double-blind, placebo-controlled drug trials reported in the Journal of the American Medical Association, the New England Journal of Medicine, and other top-of-the line medical journals—are completely in the dark about the use of natural hormones. Their use isn't taught in any medical school or promoted by any pharmaceutical company, the other major source of information for nearly all "conventional" physicians. With no multinational drug industry to pay the enormous costs, the large definitive studies that might demonstrate the efficacy and safety of natural hormones will likely never be done. Almost all doctors see only studies of the benefits and risks of Premarin,® Provera,® and other patentable "hormones," studies which the pharmaceutical industry has conducted itself or underwritten. An examination of the medical literature on HRT reveals hundreds of articles about patentable HRT for every one about natural hormone replacement.

Menopausal Myths and Misunderstandings

An unfortunate result of the use of patentable HRT and ignorance of natural hormone replacement therapy (NHR) has been the development of several myths about the medical treatment of menopause. These myths reflect a fundamental misunderstanding of the hormonal processes of menopause and reflect conventional medicine's preferred goal of "curing" menopausal symptoms rather than restoring the body's natural hormonal balance.

Myth #1: Estrogen Is a Single Hormone. In fact, estrogen is not a single hormone. The term "estrogen" is really short-hand for a group of several different but related hormones that perform the functions we normally attribute to "estrogen." Technically, it's more accurate to speak of "estrogens." In adult human women, three different natural estrogens predominate:

- Estrone (approximately 10-20% of circulating estrogens)
- Estradiol (approximately 10-20% of circulating estrogens)
- Estriol (approximately 60-80% of circulating estrogens)[4]

Under normal circumstances, hormone levels vary according to the stage of the menstrual cycle, but the amount of each hormone usually fluctuates within the proportions above.

By contrast, Premarin® is classified as a "conjugated equine estrogen." It contains primarily just one "human" estrogen, estrone (75-80%), plus equilin (6-15%), a form of estrogen found exclusively in horses (plus smaller amounts of estradiol, which is also found in humans) and two other horse estrogens. In fact, Premarin® is actually derived from the urine of pregnant mares, hence, its name. It's true that equilin can act like human estrogens

---

4. Recent laboratory investigations show that the proportion of circulating estriol may be higher than what we thought in the eighties. Please see page 127 for very recent laboratory data.

in human bodies, but it's about as "natural" in humans as any laboratory-produced, patentable hormone.

Furthermore, the proportion of estrone in Premarin® is far higher than the normal level for which the human body is designed. Premarin® is a natural hormone, all right—but natural for horses, not humans.

HUMAN ESTROGEN
- Estriol 60-80%
- Estrone 10-20%
- Estradiol 10-20%

PREMARIN®
- Estrone 75-80%
- Equilin 6-15%
- Estradiol + Others 5-19%

Most other "estrogen" prescribed by conventional medical doctors, including the estrogen patch (Estraderm®) and estrogen cream (Estrace®) are 100% estradiol, the most powerful form of estrogen, which normally comprises only about 10 to 20% of circulating human estrogens. While it's true that estradiol is a natural human hormone, unlike equilin, estradiol is still only a single type of estrogen. If the human body normally balances estradiol with estrone and estriol, there must be a good reason, even if science hasn't yet discovered what that reason may be.

Myth #2: "Estrogen" Replacement by Itself is Sufficient. This was medical gospel for many years. Fortunately, this myth is already mostly destroyed among medical doctors. Most conventional medical doctors now prescribe at least a "progestin" (a synthetic patentable drug that acts somewhat like progesterone) along with "estrogen." The risk of endometrial cancer is far too high otherwise. But the results of years of "estrogen"-only prescribing have caused many women to shy away from hormone replacement altogether.

Myth #3: Progestins=Progesterone. For exactly the same reasons that most conventional medical doctors prescribe patentable or synthetic "estrogens," they also favor patentable or synthetic progesterone substitutes known as "progestins," rather than natural progesterone. Like patentable or synthetic estrogens, progestins are capable of doing many of the same things that natural progesterone does. For example, adding a progestin (usually Provera®) to "estrogen" replacement reduces the risk of estrogen-induced endometrial cancer.

Synthetic progestins are not the same thing as natural progesterone. Unfortunately, hardly any conventional medical doctors make this distinction. They prescribe as though progestins are simply other forms of natural progesterone. It just isn't so!

As with other patentable or synthetic hormone substitutes, there's a high price to pay for the protection that progestins provide against endometrial cancer. That price includes an increased risk of heart disease, because progestins strip away some of the protection against heart disease gained from estrogen replacement. Progestins are also associated with a long list of unwanted effects, including breast tenderness, weight gain, depression, and breakthrough bleeding, to name just a few. These unwanted effects often cause women to feel so bad that they stop HRT altogether. And worse, progestins do little or nothing to help osteoporosis.

Natural progesterone is a completely different story. Because it is identical to the progesterone our bodies produce, replacement of missing progesterone with natural progesterone puts back the exact same hormone that our bodies are accustomed to. As a result, when used properly, natural progesterone protects against endometrial cancer, does not interfere with estrogen's cardiovascular protection, and has virtually no unwanted effects. And if this were not enough reason to use it, natural progesterone also can rebuild bone, even after it's been lost.

Myth #4: Estriol Is a Weak and Unimportant Estrogen. Estriol has been largely overlooked by most American physicians and pharmaceutical researchers, who have long considered it to be an inactive, or at best, a weak and unimportant metabolite of estrone and estradiol. Why go through all the trouble of putting it into a pill if you don't really need it?

This reasoning is completely wrong! As one researcher pointed out in a review of six decades of estriol research, "It would be unusual if nature produced three estrogens of which only one was utilized." Estriol is needed, and here's why.

It now appears that the primary cancer danger from synthetic HRT does not come from "unopposed" estrogen (since taking progestin or natural progesterone solves this), but from "unopposed" estradiol, estrone, and equilin. A number of scientific studies, published over four decades, have demonstrated that estriol's unique, and perhaps most important role may be to oppose the growth of cancer, including cancer promoted by estradiol and estrone, themselves. Consider these facts:

- The results of animal studies have suggested that when natural estradiol and estrone are "opposed" with estriol in normal (physiologic) proportions, the risk of cancer due to hormone replacement virtually vanishes.
- When taken by itself, even in relatively high doses, estriol does not increase endometrial proliferation.

The European medical community has been more open-minded about estriol. Doctors in Europe have accepted and prescribed it as a safe and effective alternative to 100% estradiol or Premarin® for years. They have found it especially helpful for women with disabling postmenopausal symptoms, such as vaginal thinning, painful sexual intercourse, recurrent urinary tract infections, and urinary incontinence.

Myth #5: "Estrogen" Replacement Prevents Osteoporosis. To prevent osteoporosis—the reduction in bone density that can lead to fractures of the hip, spine, and other bones in older people—women are urged to exercise, consume large quantities of calcium, and begin "estrogen" replacement. Good advice, but only a small part of the story! A fall in estrogens (and progesterone, and testosterone) can cause bones to become thinner and more brittle, but a rise in estrogen alone won't reverse this process.

"Estrogen" replacement may help slow or stop the osteoporotic process by slowing the death of bone cells. It will not, however, make bones any stronger than they were before ERT, because "estrogen" (even natural estrogen) does not stimulate the growth of new bone cells. The best way to stimulate new bone growth and make your bones stronger during and after menopause is to use natural progesterone, and possibly DHEA and testosterone as well.

Myth #6: The Body Does Not Absorb Natural Hormones Very Well. The natural estrogens—estradiol, estrone, and estriol—were first tested in the early 1930s. It was very difficult and expensive to prepare hormones then, and those that were produced tended to be very weak. As a result, oral versions of these hormones were thought to have little value for estrogen replacement, so little research was done on them. Scientists started looking for more potent (and patentable) synthetic versions of estrogen that could easily be packaged in pills, capsules, creams or skin patches. More recent research has demonstrated that natural hormones, as they are prepared today, are very well absorbed by the body and quite potent after either oral ingestion or from creams absorbed through the skin.

Myth #7: Testosterone and Other Androgens Are "Male" Hormones, and Women Do Not Need Them. We tend to think of estrogens as "female hormones," and androgens (the best known androgen is testosterone) as "male hormones." Actually, estrogens and testosterone are common to both men and women, though (obviously!) in very different proportions. Adrenal glands in both men and women (major sources of many steroid hormones) produce nearly equal amounts of androgens. Ovaries, the source of most estrogen and progesterone in women, also produce a significant amount of testosterone, even after menopause.

In some women, testosterone replacement with physiologic doses (doses that restore natural, youthful women's levels) has been shown to work like estrogens to reduce menopausal symptoms, such as hot flashes and vaginal dryness. Beyond its estrogen-like effects, though, testosterone is unmatched in its ability to increase most women's sexual arousal, desire, and number of orgasms. It can also increase bone density and enhance muscle strength.

DHEA (dehydroepiandrosterone) is another androgen important to both men and women. Like estrogen, progesterone, testosterone, and other hormones, DHEA levels decline with age, but starting considerably earlier since DHEA levels "peak" at age 25 to 30. By age 50, we have only a fraction of the DHEA we had in our late 20s. Some DHEA is metabolized into testosterone and estrogens, but unmetabolized DHEA has independent effects ranging from prevention of heart disease and cancer to weight loss.

Considerable recent scientific evidence confirms that restoring DHEA to youthful levels may help safely boost estrogen and testosterone levels by a small amount.

Myth #8: Any Synthetic Hormone Approved by the FDA Must Be Better and/or Safer Than the Natural (Unapproved) Hormone it Replaces. This one can't be serious! The FDA's been around since 1906, while natural human hormones have been around since the dawn of human history! If the FDA has approved Premarin® and Provera® for use in treating menopause, these hormones must be better and safer than natural estrogens and natural progesterone which do not have that "official stamp of approval?" As my kids say, "NOT!"

The FDA's enormously expensive drug approval process prevents rigorous scientific study of natural hormone replacement therapy, so there's (so far) no direct way to compare "HRT" and "NHR." If we don't have as much "scientific" evidence about NHR, it's because very little money has been spent to study it. So, because of ignorance and misconceptions about natural hormones combined with fear of malpractice suits, it's hard to find a physician who would argue with this myth.

The FDA has absolutely no interest in finding the best way to treat the effects of menopause (or anything else). This is not entirely the FDA's fault, since its Congressionally-mandated purpose is not to find the best treatment for anything, but only to find out if the drugs submitted to it for whatever reason meet standards of safety and efficacy.

When a Premarin,® a Provera,® or any other drug is submitted, it is evaluated solely on its own merits. It's never tested to see how it compares with its natural counterpart. The pharmaceutical companies submitting their patented drugs prefer this arrangement, because they're especially not interested in testing any alternative, natural or not. If the new drug is found to be better than an inactive placebo, and if its risk-to-benefit ratio is judged to be within acceptable limits, it is approved; if not, it is not. No other comparative testing is done.

This system of drug approval leaves a huge gap into which excellent, and often superior, substances, like natural estrogens, natural progesterone, and hundreds of other valuable natural therapies, fall unless people and doctors go to the trouble to evaluate them on their own.

The FDA "stamp of approval" on Premarin® or Provera® tells you nothing at all about how good these drugs are compared with natural hormones. To find this out, we either need to do large, expensive, long-term clinical trials comparing the two or, more realistically, read the scientific literature on both and make up our own minds. If we do the latter, it's obvious that natural hormones are the best choice.

Why You Should Consider
Natural Hormone Replacement

For the majority of women who have used Premarin,® Provera,® or other patentable or synthetic hormones to ease the symptoms of early menopause, the results have been mostly positive. But in the absence of any "medically accepted" alternatives to these drugs for the last four decades, women have been asked to gamble with their lives, accepting a small risk of cancer in return for a larger chance of preventing atherosclerosis, osteoporosis, and possibly, senility and memory loss. Natural hormone replacement therapy (NHR) greatly improves women's odds of "winning" that gamble.

NHR is the next logical step in menopausal hormone replacement therapy. The concept of replacing hormones with identical hormones in the correct proportions at the correct time makes obvious sense. How could the human species have survived if normal levels of every woman's reproductive hormones predisposed her to fatal disease during her fertile years? If natural human hormones increased women's cancer risk much at all, the human species would probably have gone extinct long ago.

For some, close observation of nature and creation is reason enough to switch from HRT to NHR. For those who need "proof," scientific evidence continues to build in favor of using a balanced combination of natural estrogens (approximately 10-20% estradiol, 10-20% estrone, and 60-80% estriol, plus natural progesterone, and in many cases, DHEA and testosterone) in place of patented, laboratory designed estradiol alone or horse estrogen plus a progestin, and possibly synthetic methyltestosterone.

The advantages of NHR for menopausal and perimenopausal women are now quite clear. They include all the well-known benefits of HRT and more, with very few of the unwanted effects and risks associated with the man-made variety:

- Prevention of osteoporosis & restoration of bone strength
- Reduced hot flashes & reduced vaginal dryness/thinning
- Better maintenance of muscle mass & strength
- Protection against heart disease & stroke
- Improved cholesterol levels
- Reduced risk of endometrial cancer & breast cancer
- Reduced risk of depression
- Improved sleep & better mood, concentration & memory
- Prevention of senility & Alzheimer's disease
- Improved libido (sex drive)
- Many fewer unwanted effects than with synthetic hormones

Beyond Estrogens
and Progesterone

For many women, natural estrogens and progesterone may only be the start of natural hormone replacement. Estrogens and progesterone are just part of a complex and closely interlinked hormonal system that includes many other hormones, including testosterone, DHEA, pregnenolone, and melatonin, to name just a few.

Like estrogens and progesterone, many of these hormones have also been found to decline with age. And like estrogens and progesterone, restoring many of them to normal levels with natural replacement versions can have a remarkably revitalizing effect on everything from our hearts and immune systems to our moods, energy, and libido.

In the rest of this book, the benefits and drawbacks of both natural and synthetic hormone replacement will be compared. You'll read why natural alternatives are clearly the best choice. You'll also find answers to questions like, "Are they really that good? And that safe?" "Do I need to get my doctor to prescribe them for me?" "Where can I buy natural hormones? The health food store?

The pharmacy?"

In short, you'll find all the information you need to evaluate all the known options and, should you choose hormone replacement, to choose wisely.

CHAPTER 2

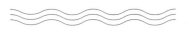

Hormones of
the Menstrual Cycle

AS A MALE, I APOLOGIZE in advance for having the nerve to explain menstrual cycle hormones to a woman! If you find this chapter unnecessary or boring, please feel free to skip to the next chapter. However, a brief review about hormones may be a help in understanding the logic of NHR, especially its timing. If you decide to skip this chapter for now—you can always review the material later if you need to—please go right on to Chapter 3.

In order to understand what happens during perimenopause and menopause, and how hormone replacement works, let's review some basic information about the normal menstrual cycle. The story of menstruation and menopause is really the story of the ovaries, the uterus and the pituitary gland.

Within each ovary are thousands of tiny sacs called follicles. At the time a woman has her first period, she may have as many as 500,000 follicles, each of which is filled with eggs. Usually, early in each menstrual cycle, just one of these eggs begins to "ripen." (It's one of the wonders of nature and creation that only one egg "knows" its time has arrived, and the rest just "wait 'til next month.") Around mid-cycle, the follicle bursts open, and the ripened egg passes into the fallopian tube, which leads to the uterus. This process is called *ovulation*. If it meets sperm along the way, the egg may be fertilized, and the resulting fertilized egg soon begins to divide and differentiate into multiple cells while continuing its journey to the uterus.

In the meantime, the uterus has been preparing to welcome and nurture the newly fertilized egg since the end of the last menstrual period. The lining of the uterus (the endometrium) has become thicker and enriched with blood and nutrients, so when the fertilized egg reaches its destination, it can easily implant itself into the uterine wall and begin to grow into an embryo, a fetus, and eventually, an infant.

If the egg is not fertilized, it still continues its journey into the uterus. In the absence of a hormonal message that fertilization has occurred, however, the uterus ends its preparations for pregnancy and discards the endometrial lining it has built up, as well as the extra blood and nutrients it has amassed.

This familiar event is known by a number of names: menstruation, menstrual bleeding, "my period," "the curse," and many others. In addition to signaling a woman that she is healthy and not pregnant, regular menstruation is also a sign that conception is still possible in the future. Once menstruation starts to lose its regularity (usually every 26-28 days), it probably means menopause is approaching, and the remaining fertile days are numbered. When periods stop altogether, menopause has arrived.

The amazing regularity of the menstrual cycle is primarily due to a balance of four hormones:
- Estrogens
- Progesterone
- Follicle Stimulating Hormone (FSH)
- Luteinizing Hormone (LH)

Although in this book, estrogen sometimes appears in the singular for the sake of convenience, remember that estrogen is really three hormones: estrone, estradiol, and estriol. FSH and LH are also known as *pituitary gonadotropins* (hormones secreted by the pituitary gland which stimulate the "gonads"—women's ovaries and men's testicles).

Of course, menstrual cycles continue for approximately 40 years with no real beginning or end, but it's convenient to speak of the first day of menstruation as the end of one cycle and the beginning of the next. Figure 2.1 illustrates in schematic form the multiple events that occur simultaneously during the menstrual cycle.

Days 1-5: Estrogen falls, FSH rises. Menstrual bleeding begins on Day 1 of the cycle and lasts approximately 5 days. During the last few days prior to Day 1, a sharp fall in the levels of estrogen

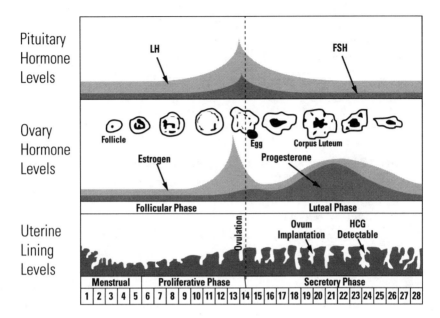

Fig. 2.1: Events of the Normal Menstrual Cycle

and progesterone signals the uterus that pregnancy has not occurred during this cycle. This signal results in a shedding of the endometrial lining of the uterus.

Since high levels of estrogen suppress the secretion of FSH (a "negative feedback loop"), the drop in estrogen now permits the level of FSH to rise. As its name implies, follicle stimulating hormone stimulates follicle development. By Day 5 to 7 of the cycle, one of these follicles responds to FSH stimulation more than the others and becomes dominant. As it does so, it begins secreting large amounts of estrogen.

Days 6-14: Estrogen rises, FSH falls. The large amount of estrogen secreted by the follicle during this phase of the menstrual cycle has several important effects:

- It stimulates the endometrial lining of the uterus to become thicker and enriched in preparation for implantation of the fertilized egg.

- It suppresses the further secretion of FSH ("negative feedback").
- At about mid-cycle (Day 14), it helps stimulate a large and sudden release of luteinizing hormone. This LH surge, which is accompanied by a transient rise in body temperature, is a sign that ovulation is about to happen.
- The LH surge causes the follicle to rupture and expel the egg into the fallopian tube.

Days 14-28: Estrogen and progesterone secretion first rise, then fall. After the follicle ruptures, its walls collapse, and it is now known as the *corpus luteum.* Immediately after ovulation, the corpus luteum begins secreting large amounts of progesterone, which also helps prepare the endometrial lining for implantation of the fertilized egg. If the egg is fertilized, a small amount of the hormone called *human chorionic gonadotrophin (HCG)* is released. HCG, which can be detected as early as seven days after fertilization, is the basis for the early pregnancy tests that have become so popular.

HCG keeps the corpus luteum viable, so it can continue pumping out estrogen and progesterone, which, in turn, keep the endometrial lining intact. By about Week 6 to 8 of gestation, the newly formed placenta takes over the secretion of progesterone.

If the egg is not fertilized, the corpus luteum starts to "run out of gas" (actually, it starts to run out of hormone), causing the levels of estrogen and progesterone to drop. Without these hormones to support it, the uterus soon sheds its lining, and menstruation begins. In addition, with no estrogen to suppress it, FSH levels again start to rise. Thus, one cycle ends and another begins.

What Happens During Perimenopause and Menopause?

During the decades when the menstrual top is spinning along smoothly, the key to its flawless rotation is balance—specifically, the hormonal balance among estrogen, progesterone, FSH, and LH. As estrogen rises, FSH falls. As estrogen falls, FSH rises. In perimenopause, the top starts to go slightly out of balance; estrogen and/or progesterone cycle at lower than usual levels, and FSH and/or LH are somewhat higher than before, while still cycling. After menopause, the typical pattern would be continually high levels of FSH and continually low levels of estrogen and progesterone.

The follicles remaining in the ovaries of a perimenopausal woman are generally less sensitive to stimulation by FSH than the ones that preceded them. Increasingly, there will be cycles in which no follicle develops fully, and eventually, cycles in which no follicle develops at all. For most of the perimenopause, normal and abnormal cycles tend to be intermixed. One month a follicle will develop normally, and other months, with increasing frequency, it will not.

When a follicle fails to develop properly, it secretes less estrogen. The low level of estrogen cannot fully suppress the secretion of FSH by the pituitary gland. So, as estrogen levels fall, FSH levels rise. If estrogen levels are sufficiently low, they may fail to trigger the LH surge that's supposed to rupture the follicle, and the egg isn't released. This is termed an anovulatory cycle (a cycle without ovulation).

If the follicle doesn't rupture, the corpus luteum cannot form, and consequently, progesterone cannot be released at the appropriate time. The lack of normal amounts of estrogen gives rise to all the familiar discomforts of estrogen deficiency, from hot flushes and insomnia to depression and palpitations. In the long run, heart disease and osteoporosis may follow.

The decline of estrogen and progesterone, which may happen before the perimenopause, signals the uterus to shed its endometrial lining prematurely. This results in a general shortening of the length of the cycles, and often, the timing of estrogen and progesterone decline varies from month to month, resulting in irregular cycles. Shorter cycles, irregular cycles, or both are often the first signs that the perimenopause has started.

Androgens, like testosterone, also decline during this period, but curiously, at a much slower rate than estrogen and progesterone in many women. The ovaries continue to secrete testosterone even after menopause. As we shall see in the chapters that follow, it's possible to keep the menstrual top spinning with a minimum of wobbling even after the ovaries have started to shut down. Applying the natural hormones—estrone, estradiol, estriol, and progesterone—at the appropriate times in the appropriate amounts mimics the natural ebb and flow of the body's own hormones, and the body reacts as though the ovaries were still functioning normally.

During the perimenopausal years, appropriate natural hormone replacement (NHR) can relieve symptoms and continue the prior pattern of menstrual bleeding. Once "menopause age" (which varies from family to family) arrives, quantities of NHR can be reduced sufficiently to eliminate menstrual bleeding while still giving protection against cardiovascular disease, osteoporosis, and loss of mental function.

Actually, even more hormones are involved in the normal menstrual cycle than those mentioned above. These include "releasing hormones" for FSH and LH, and likely, others that science hasn't yet discovered or fully described. But certain "hormones" are totally and conspicuously absent from the human menstrual cycle: conjugated equine estrogens (Premarin®), medroxyprogesterone (Provera®) or other "progestins" or "progestogens," and methyltestosterone. Not one patentable molecule is a part of any woman's normal menstrual cycling!

Escape From
"Menopause Hell"

Stella Osborne had a relatively typical problem with "perimenopausal hormone wobbling." That's not how she saw it, though.

"I think I'm going through menopause hell," she declared. "For the last year-and-a-half, maybe a little longer, I can never tell when or if my period's going to show up. Sometimes it's really light, a 'drip day' or two, then nothing. Sometimes, I'm standing there ... usually in the middle of a meeting ... and it's flood city! With no warning! I feel like I should use two tampons whenever I go out whether I need them or not, just in case.

"For awhile, I thought I'd finally stopped ... nothing for five months. Then, for no particular reason, I had two practically normal ones in a row. Then, back to who knows what? And, if this bleeding weren't bad enough, I've been … well, a real witch (and I cleaned that word up) at home with absolutely no warning at all."

"Sometimes, I even surprise myself. The depression and mood swings are awful, and many nights I can't get any sleep. I don't want to take Premarin® or Provera.® I read the warnings with my friend's prescriptions. I've heard that you prescribe natural hormones. Can natural hormones help me?"

I tried not to smile. "That's what they were doing until one-and-a-half years ago, right?"

She broke into a wide smile herself. "When you put it that way, it was a bit of a dumb question, wasn't it?"

"No questions are dumb questions when it involves getting our health in order. Now let's see … you're 46?"

"Yes."

"Do you have any idea when your mother or any older sisters went through menopause?"

"No older sisters, but Mom says 52 or 53. I'm starting early."

"If that's the case, then it seems logical to use enough natural hormone replacement to maintain your normal menstrual bleeding pattern until about Mom's menopause age, and then reduce the quantity to enough to protect your heart, arteries, bones, brain … and for that matter, all the rest of you … without producing menstrual bleeding. But having the larger quantity of natural hormones until at least Mom's menopause time is probably healthier."

"OK. I wasn't looking forward to menstrual periods until I'm 80 or whatever."

"Actually, that is another 'school of thought' in natural hormone replacement."

"What, periods until 80 years old?" She looked surprised.

"Yes. The theory is that normal monthly loss of the endometrium is healthier."

"You don't subscribe to that theory?"

"The past 30 years of 'hormone' replacement therapy for

women after menopause—even with patentable 'estrogen' and 'progestins' or incomplete 'estrogen' and 'progestin'—have been done without regular cyclic bleeding. As long as even 'progestin' was used, there wasn't any extra uterine cancer risk. That's the most important data we have.

"Secondly, to be practical, most women react just as you did: 'Excuse me, but I'd rather not have menstrual bleeding until I'm 93, please.'"

"Are you sure there'll be enough hormone at that age to do the job?" she asked.

"Yes. Tests such as bone scans confirming an increase in bone density after age 70 have convinced me of that."

"Good. I'll worry about that when the time comes. For now, give me the natural hormone replacement, and I'll just keep "cycling away" normally and regularly, I hope, for the next few years!"

Her prescriptions did just that. During the perimenopausal years, appropriate natural hormone replacement therapy (NHR) can (and usually does) relieve symptoms and continue the prior pattern of menstrual bleeding. NHR also reliably banishes "witchiness," mood swings, depression, insomnia, and other symptoms of insufficient hormones. As I explained to Mrs. Osborne, once "menopause age" (which varies from family to family) arrives, the quantities of natural hormones can be reduced sufficiently to eliminate menstrual bleeding while still giving protection against cardiovascular disease, osteoporosis, and loss of mental function.

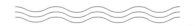

CHAPTER 3

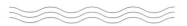

Hormones: Patentable, Natural, or Natural for Horses?

ASK MOST MEDICAL DOCTORS about natural hormone replacement therapy, and they'll probably tell you about "conjugated estrogens" derived from horse urine. What they likely won't mention is natural hormone replacement therapy (NHR). Not that they think there's anything wrong with NHR. More than likely, they're confused (or just haven't thought) about just which hormones are truly "natural" for their patients.

Even as a medical doctor practicing "natural medicine" in the 1970s, I just hadn't thought about natural hormone replacement much at all. My medical school had emphasized the use of Premarin® while telling us it was "natural." Hormones identical to human hormones weren't available anyway, so I didn't worry much about it until 1982, when a woman I was working with told me Premarin® "just didn't feel quite right" and asked if there was an alternative. What should have been obvious before then dawned: Why not just duplicate what Nature and Creation intended anyway?

Surprisingly, (or on reflection, perhaps not), textbooks of gynecology and obstetrics dutifully mentioned all the naturally occurring hormones but completely neglected to recommend their use in treatment. A few clinical testing laboratories were kind enough to send me their latest information about normal levels of each circulating estrogen (after asking politely, "What do you need that information for?"). Their "lab normals" showed the proportions of each of the three natural estrogens (approximately ... but more about that later) as given in the last chapter.

In the early 1980s, compounding pharmacists (pharmacists who put together doctors' prescriptions "from scratch" instead of just

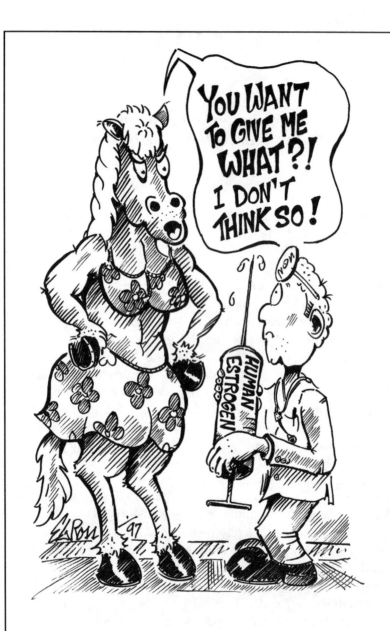

If the shoe were on the other hoof

NATURAL HORMONE REPLACEMENT IN MEDIEVAL TIMES

NATURAL HORMONE REPLACEMENT therapy isn't a new idea. According to Joseph Needham (*Science and Civilization in China,* Volume 5, Part 5, Cambridge University Press, 1983), Taoist physicians made and used preparations of human urine solids containing sex steroids from at least the 11th century onward, and possibly as long as 2,000 years ago.

In many cases, these preparations were used specifically to promote longevity and restore sexual vigor and potency in both sexes. Urine of boys and/or girls in their teens or early twenties was often specified. Of course, urine of individuals at these ages contains the largest amount of sex-specific hormones and hormone metabolites.

counting out premanufactured pills) weren't as popular or numerous as they are today. Ed Thorpe, my pharmacist friend at Kripps Pharmacy, Vancouver, British Columbia, volunteered to compound (to my prescription) estrone, estradiol, and estriol in identical-to-natural quantities and proportions. This combination later became known as "triple estrogen" or "Tri-Est."

Meanwhile, Dr. John Lee of Sebastopol, California, had started researching and prescribing natural progesterone in 1979, and it had become available in most compounding pharmacies. With triple estrogen and natural progesterone, the major elements of NHR were in place.

In 1997, whether a hormone is said to be "natural" or "synthetic" depends as much on marketing as on science. While everyone will agree that the hormones we're born with are natural, the picture gets much muddier when these natural hormones are replaced with versions that come from laboratories or horses' ovaries. If we apply informed reason to the subject, the following categories may help cut through all the confusion:

Natural Hormones. The hormones the human body normally produces, estrone, estradiol, estriol, progesterone, and testosterone, are all natural hormones. It may seem paradoxical at first that the "natural" estrone, estradiol, and estriol used for natural hormone replacement do not come from humans, as they did hundreds and even thousands of years ago [see box on previous page].

Today, these hormones for NHR get their start from the wild yam *(Diascorea composita)* which is rich in "precursor" molecules easily converted by biochemists into other molecules that are identical in every way to "natural" estrogens, progesterone, testosterone, and other hormones.

How can a hormone which got its start in a vegetable and was converted in a test tube be considered "natural" in a human female? When describing replacement hormones, the word "natural" is used to refer to the structure of the hormone molecule, not its source. When analyzed biochemically, the molecules of estrogens, progesterone, and other hormones produced from wild yam precursor molecules are found to be absolutely indistinguishable from those the human body produces itself. Thus the crucial variable defining "natural" is not the origin of the hormone but its chemical structure.[1]

Patentable Hormones. The word patentable usually suggests "artificial" or not found in nature, and with hormones, it is no different. Patentable "hormones" are typically those, like ethinyl estradiol, which scientists have altered slightly from the original estrogen to create a molecule that looks something like a natural estrogen but, in fact, is different from any estrogen ever found in nature or creation. This is the same strategy pharmaceutical industry scientists use to create "progestins" designed to mimic the actions of natural progesterone.

---

1. You can't increase your estrogen levels by eating wild yam because the human physiology does not include the requisite enzymes for converting the hormone precursors in these vegetables to estrogen. There are other vegetables you can eat that may help raise your estrogen levels, however. The most common of these are soy products, such as tofu, miso, soy sauces, and others, which contain chemicals called phytoestrogens. It is thought that Asian women suffer less from the symptoms of menopause and perimenopause than Western women because of the extremely high soy content of their diet. See Chapter 11 for more on this important subject.

When a substance such as horse urine concentrate cannot legally be patented because it occurs somewhere in nature, a "process patent" may still be granted that covers the way in which the material is collected or processed. Of course, patents eventually expire, but I'll refer to even previously patented "hormones" as "patentable."

If It Acts Like a Hormone ...

Much of the confusion surrounding the definition of natural hormones arises when we're careless (sometimes intentionally, sometimes not) with the definition of a hormone. According to *Dorland's Illustrated Medical Dictionary,* the classical definition of a hormone is "a chemical substance, produced in the body by an organ or cells of a certain organ, which has a specific regulatory effect on the activity of a certain organ." *Dorland's* goes on to point out that this definition has been loosened (by some) in recent years to apply to any substance that may act like a hormone, even though it may not be produced in the body by the specialized glands that normally produce and secrete hormones.

This broadened definition of a hormone opens the door to using all kinds of other substances as hormone "replacements." Some of these substances may not be hormones in the original sense of the word, and they may differ in chemical structure in one or more important aspects from the natural hormones they're intended to replace. Nevertheless, they may act like natural hormones in many ways.

This can lead to a mind set that says, "If it acts like an estrogen (or progesterone), it must be an estrogen (or progesterone)." Since the early 1900s, pharmaceutical companies have worked very hard to sell us all this concept since it allows them to sell enormously profitable patentable substances under the "hormone" label. (Unfortunately, these huge profits from patentable "hormones" have come at the expense of increased risk of adverse effects in women's bodies.)

It also encourages the use of other "naturally occurring" hormones, like conjugated equine estrogens (Premarin®), in human women, even though Nature evolved them over millions of years to fit the unique physiology of the female horse.

Well, one might ask, if it acts like an estrogen (or progesterone), why not use it as an estrogen? What difference does it really make, as long as it reduces perimenopausal discomforts and prevents the long-term consequences of estrogen (and progesterone) depletion after menopause? The short answer is that it makes a big difference, not only in the way these substances produce their hormone-like effects, but also, and perhaps more importantly, from the way the cells of our bodies interact with them.

So get a cup of tea (herbal, of course) or coffee (organically grown, naturally decaffeinated), relax, and bear with me, as the next section is likely to be the most technical. Sorry, but please hang in there; once you understand this part, no one will ever be able to fool you with "patentable" hormones (or for that matter other "patentable" substances) ever again!

How Hormones Carry Vital Chemical Messages

A hormone is a "chemical messenger." Once released from its point of origin, usually a gland, a hormone travels throughout the body by floating through the blood stream—sometimes for great distances, and sometimes for only a few millimeters—until it encounters a "target" cell containing a specially shaped hormone receptor.

Think of a target cell as a restaurant with a neon sign on the roof flashing, "Gourmet Food, All You Can Eat! … Members Only." The "hormone receptor" is a specific door into the restaurant.

Think of hormones as two-ended keys, one end labeled "R," the other end labeled "E." To enter the restaurant, the "Hormone A Key" has to open locked "Receptor Door A" using the "R" (for receptor) end. Once the hormone "unlocks" the restaurant door, it signals the kitchen to spring into action, churning out the specialty dish(es) "Hormone A" regularly orders up.

Target cells sensitive to all kinds of hormones are located all over the body. If a target cell happens to be a muscle cell, it may contract when an appropriate hormone comes for lunch; a gland cell may secrete (or suppress the secretion of) another hormone. (Remember high levels of estrogen "shutting off" production of the hormone FSH?)

Under ordinary conditions, only the "R" end of the "Hormone A Key" can open "Receptor Lock A." However, there are circumstances when a drug molecule may be shaped enough like the "R" end of "Hormone A Key" that it, too, can fit the lock on "Receptor Door A."

While the drug molecule may look a lot like "Hormone A," it certainly doesn't act the same once it unlocks the receptor door. It may order up "Hormone A's" favorite food from the menu, but its appetite may be bigger or smaller—demanding that the kitchen churn out more or less food. It may order up other items from the menu as well, and it may not know when to leave.

Remember the other end of the Hormone Key, the "E" end? It's not meant to fit the receptor door lock (that's the "R" end). The "E" end is designed to fit into locks on certain specific chemicals called *enzymes,* which hormones often encounter in their travels. When the "E" end of the Hormone Key comes upon an "E" lock on an enzyme, the enzyme goes to work changing the hormone key in some way. Often the result is to change (or "morph," as our kids say) the original hormone into different molecules known as hormone metabolites. These metabolites may be more or less active than the original hormone.

Unfortunately, many drugs (and even many environmental pollutants) mimic the physiologic effects of hormones. These drugs may have an "R" end similar enough to the "R" end of the "Hormone A Key" to unlock "Receptor Door A." But because the other end of their molecular "keys" aren't at all like the "E" end of "Hormone A Key," the body may lack enzymes with the correctly shaped "lock" to process them properly and/or completely. As a result, these imitation "hormone" drugs usually have unwanted effects; they may also be more or less potent; and their effects may be longer- or shorter-lasting.

A prime example is equilin, one of the ingredients in horse estrogen (Premarin®). Compare the molecular skeleton of equilin with those of the natural estrogens (estradiol, estrone, and estriol) in Figure 3.1.

It doesn't take a biochemist to see that all the molecules (except di-ethylstilbestrol) have very similar chemical structures. They are

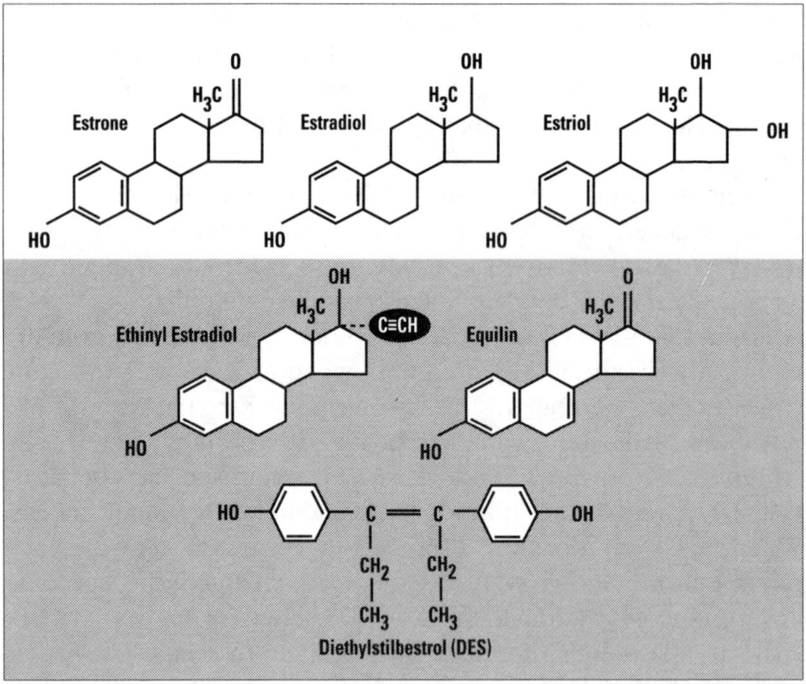

Fig. 3.1: Structure of the Natural Estrogens Compared to Some Others.

all built on a basic foundation that reflects their common ancestry as members of the steroid family. It is this basic steroid structure plus very specific additions to that "steroid foundation" that allows them to produce their "estrogenic" effects.

Just as important as the similarities of these estrogenic molecules, though, are their differences. These subtle differences are important because they determine the way the molecules interact, not only with estrogenic receptors, but also with those enzymes that, among other things, help neutralize and dispose of them after they have finished their work.

As described in Chapters 1 and 2, estrone, estradiol, and estriol are the three natural estrogens all women are born with and produce in large quantities throughout their reproductive lives. Women are also born with the enzymes they need to metabolize (i.e., chemically change, neutralize, and/or dispose of) these natural hormones, so they exert their desired effects in just the right amount for just the right time and then quietly leave. The catch is that these enzymes may not necessarily process patentable hormone molecules in exactly the same way or to precisely the same degree.

Take equilin, for example. (On second thought, don't *take* it, please! Let's just use it as an example.) Horses have all the enzymes they need to process equilin, but humans do not. Because it occurs naturally in horses, equilin is widely referred to in conventional medical circles as a "natural" estrogen suitable for humans. Thanks to decades of excellent promotion by the pharmaceutical industry and a lack of contrary information in conventional medical journals (which are largely supported by advertising from those same pharmaceutical companies), many doctors have bought this fiction.

But the use of horse estrogen by human women can lead to serious problems. As two leading reproductive physiologists have pointed out: "Levels [of equilin] can remain elevated for 13 weeks or more post-treatment due to storage and slow release from adipose [fat] tissue. In addition, metabolism of equilin to equelenin and 17-hydroxy-equilenin may contribute greatly to the estrogen stimulatory effect of [conjugated estrogen] therapy. *For this reason, conjugated estrogens are, strictly speaking, not natural to human beings."* (Italics added for emphasis.)

Translated into everyday language, this reinforces the fact that, like having four hooves, a mane, and a strong back, equine females also differ somewhat from human females in the intrinsic nature of their hormones. (Doesn't it seem strange to be repeating this point? Even small children know that women differ from mares ... but I've decided to repeat it anyway in case you give this book to your doctor.) Horses have no trouble metabolizing horse hormones, but the human body lacks the enzymes to do the job properly. As a result, equilin produces estrogenic effects that are much, much more potent and much longer lasting than those produced by natural human estrogens. It has been estimated that horse estrogens are as much as eight times more potent than natural human estrogens in the human body.

The farther away we get from the natural human estrogen molecules, the greater the problems become. Ethinyl estradiol, for example, is a completely synthetic form of the basic estrogen molecule that was designed to be highly effective when taken by mouth (as well as to be patentable). Consequently, it is the most common form of estrogen used in birth control pills. Like most man-made versions of natural molecules, this apparent advantage has a serious down side. Because ethinyl estradiol is not metabolized in the liver the way natural estradiol is, it hangs around in the body far longer. It may be as much as 1,000 times more potent than its natural counterpart!

Di-ethylstilbesterol (DES) is even worse. Notice (in Figure 3.1) that the DES molecule looks quite different from the natural estrogen molecules, human or horse. There is a good reason for this. While all the other forms of estrogen shown are at least members of the steroid family, DES is not even a distant cousin. It is a *nonsteroidal* compound that just happens to act like an estrogen in some ways. DES was cooked up by biochemists in an attempt to find a patentable drug that mimicked the actions of estrogen, not to replace missing natural estrogen. You can't get any more synthetic than that. (Another nonsteroidal chemical you may have heard of that acts like an estrogen in some ways is the pesticide DDT.)

When DES was first synthesized back in the late 1930s, it was promoted as a cheap and plentiful form of estrogen. Seen as a true milestone in the days when natural hormones were scarce and costly, it was given to many pregnant women during their first trimesters to help prevent miscarriages.

It was not until decades later that observant researchers noticed that far too many of the daughters of women who took DES during their pregnancy were developing vaginal and cervical cancer. The reason? Apparently, a developing infant lacks the enzymes to properly dispose of DES, so the drug accumulates in the body, free to exert its carcinogenic effects.

Where Do Hormones Come From?

Hormones, even natural ones, are made, not born. Like any other molecules our bodies make, our bodies create the natural hormones we need from nutrients, with the help of enzymes. Estrogens, androgens, progesterone, and other members of the

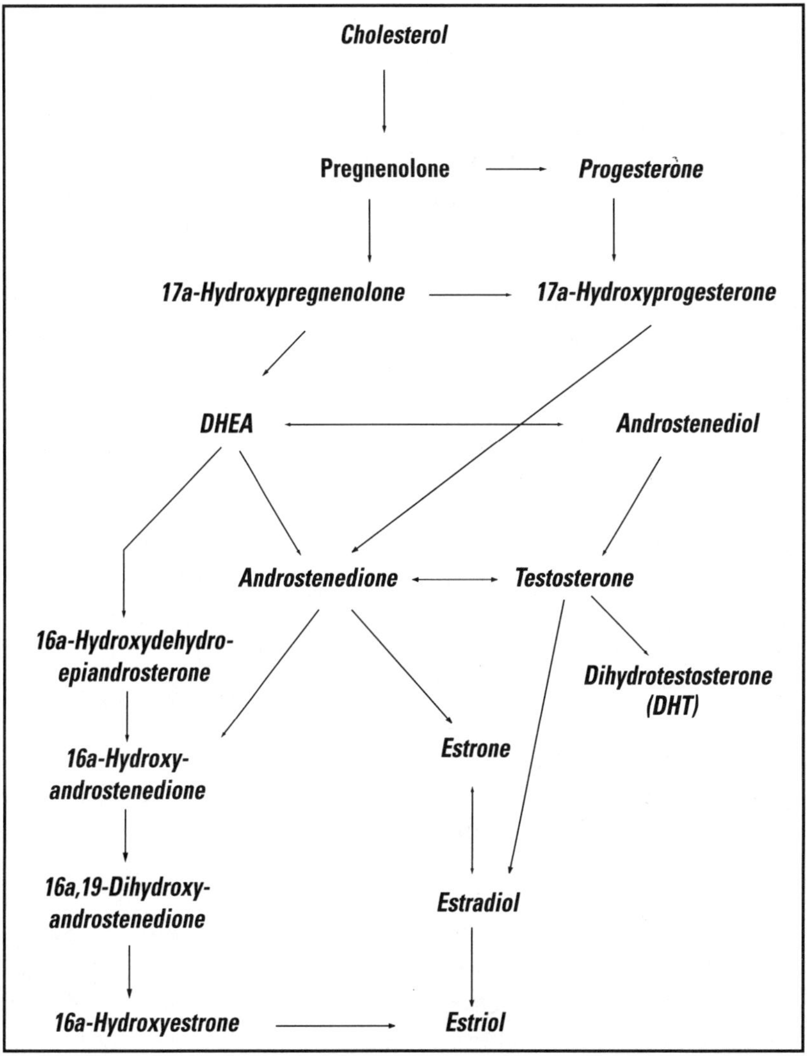

Fig. 3.2: Steroid Family Tree

steroid family can all trace their roots back to a single "ancestor" molecule. You may have heard of this precursor. It's a fatty substance known as cholesterol (Fig. 3.2).

Although it doesn't get much good press these days, cholesterol is actually a vital substance our bodies require for (among other reasons) producing the full range of steroid hormones. No cholesterol, no estrogen, no testosterone. Although the body produces much of the cholesterol it needs in the liver, it is not uncommon for people who go on extremely low-fat, low-cholesterol diets to find that their hormonal balance is disturbed.

As you can see in Figure 3.2, the Steroid Family Tree begins with cholesterol, some of which is converted to the hormone pregnenolone. Pregnenolone, in turn, begets both progesterone and DHEA. Some progesterone and some DHEA are both converted into androstenedione, a major precursor (by separate "pathways") of both estrone and testosterone. Testosterone, the best-known of the "male hormones," can be converted to the "female hormone" estradiol.

Estrone and estradiol have an interesting relationship in that some estrone is also changed into estradiol, and some estradiol is changed back to estrone. Most of the estrone and estradiol the body produces is quickly converted to estriol, but just to keep things interesting, some estriol can be produced from DHEA or androstenedione without involving estrone or estradiol at all!

(If this is confusing, don't feel bad. Only full-time steroid researchers have all this memorized, and they're the first to admit there may be metabolic pathways and interrelationships among all these steroids that no one yet knows about.)

For a long time, medical doctors and researchers have looked at all these relationships and dismissed estriol as "just an unimportant metabolite" of estrone and estradiol. (From the 1930s to the late 1980s, medical doctors dismissed DHEA in the same way as an "unimportant metabolite.") This view was reinforced by the observation that estriol appeared to be less actively "estrogenic" than the other two. (Inactive or less active metabolites are quite common in the body.) Those women who have used estriol know well that estriol is far from inactive. In fact, studies have shown that estriol also helps neutralize still-active estradiol and estrone by as much as 30% by competing with them for estrogen receptor sites, thus preventing them from stimulating these sites.

Why Natural Hormones are Better
The extraordinary balance among estradiol, estrone, estriol and

the other steroid hormones is maintained by a dazzlingly complex array of enzymes and feedback loops. Thus, if the level of one hormone is too high, the system can usually compensate by reducing the production of that hormone, enhancing its metabolism, and/or increasing the production of other enzymes and hormones to oppose it.

If you add large amounts of one or more estrogens to this system, the delicate balance is likely to be disrupted. For example, there may be insufficient enzymes to metabolize the excess hormone completely or properly, leaving free hormone or active metabolites to hang around longer than they should. This may induce unhealthy or dangerous changes, such as excess growth of endometrial tissue, which may eventually lead to cancer.

This was dramatically demonstrated in a study of equilin metabolism in endometrial tissue taken from postmenopausal women. The researchers found that the equilin is converted into three metabolites, one of which (17 ß-dihydroequilin) is *eight times more potent* than the parent compound for inducing endometrial growth, a possible precursor to cancer.

Keeping the Human Machine Running

The human body is a finely tuned biological machine in which all the parts are designed to work together in perfect harmony. No mechanic is his right mind would put Ford parts into a GM engine because he knows that, while some parts may look somewhat alike and function in roughly the same way, putting them together is much more likely to lead to engine malfunction or breakdown.

It's no different with hormones. When you introduce a substance into the body that the body is not prepared to handle, you're almost always asking for trouble. This risk is especially high when that substance acts like a hormone, and you take it over a long period of time. The lesson is quite simple: Replace "human parts" with human parts (even if those "parts" are tiny molecules), and the human machine is likely to keep on running a lot longer.

It's a shame most doctors don't possess the same common sense that the average auto mechanic does.

ONE MORE REASON TO AVOID HORSE ESTROGENS

IT'S BAD ENOUGH THAT HORSE estrogens can cause problems in the human physiology, but these hormones cause problems for horses, as well. Actually, it's not the hormones themselves that cause problems for the horses, but the way we humans collect them.

Recall that these hormones are derived from the urine of pregnant mares. While this may sound innocuous enough, in order to collect horse urine on a scale that makes production profitable, as many 75,000 to 80,000 pregnant mares must be confined in tiny stalls not much bigger than the horse under conditions that have raised serious alarm among people concerned with the welfare of these animals.

For most of their 11-month pregnancy, the mares live on restricted fluid intake (so as not to dilute the urine), are allowed no exercise, and may not even be allowed to lie down. After they give birth, they are allowed only a few months to pasture with their foals before they are reimpregnated to begin another round of urine production.

Even if horse estrogen were the only way women could replace their own missing estrogen, resorting to this kind of cruelty would be questionable. But given the many superior replacement hormone options available today, both natural and artificial, there would seem to be no reason to continue this barbaric practice.

Perhaps medical doctors are beginning to get the message. In a recent issue of the *Journal of Medical Ethics,* the author stated, "I determine that there is *prima facie* evidence to suggest that mares may suffer and that prescription of equine HRT (instead of synthetic estrogen-estriol) would therefore have to be justified in terms of either offering greater benefits to the women or offering greater value for money to the health service. I find that there is no substantial evidence to suggest that equine HRT offers unique advantages over and above estriol."*

* Cox, ID. Should a doctor prescribe hormone replacement therapy which has been manufactured from mare's urine? *J Med Ethics.* 1996;22: 199-204.

C H A P T E R 4

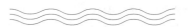

Relieving Common Menopausal Symptoms

NOT EVEN NATURAL HORMONE replacement therapy (NHR) can make a woman young again, but restoring sex hormones to more youthful levels can bring about remarkable improvements in how young she feels, how well her mind and body function, and how long she lives. Often, the appearance of women who use hormone replacement is more youthful than women who don't. In this chapter and subsequent chapters, we will examine in more detail the benefits—and risks—of hormone replacement therapy, natural and otherwise.

The only way to achieve these benefits with minimal worry about increasing the risk of cancer is to use *natural* hormones in natural quantities and proportions. As we will see, the risks associated with patentable hormones make conventional HRT a needlessly dangerous option.

No More Hot Flashes, Vaginal Pain, or Other Symptoms

For most women, the approach of menopause is signaled by unpleasant symptoms: hot flashes, night sweats, vaginal dryness, irritability, mood swings, and increased anxiety and depression. It was primarily to treat these symptoms (and other more unusual ones) that the first ERT regimens were developed and have been extremely successful.

Not surprisingly, most of the published studies on the role of "estrogen" replacement in treating common menopausal symptoms have employed patentable "estrogens," usually conjugated equine estrogens (Premarin®). Sometimes 100% estradiol was given, but hardly ever in combination with estrone, and certainly not combined with estriol.

Though effective for menopausal symptoms, these "estrogens" and "progestins" are essentially *illegal aliens* in the human body. They've managed to sneak across the body's border, usually penetrating through the gastrointestinal (GI) tract after being swallowed as a pill or capsule, or getting absorbed through the skin, suspended in a cream or embedded in a patch. They mingle with the body's native hormones and perform many of the functions of native hormones, but they don't speak the body's language well, and they don't have the proper molecular *credentials* to interact with all the appropriate enzymes.

These "hormones"—drugs, really—have been chosen largely for their ability to get into the human body and to mimic the ability of natural *human* estrogens to prevent hot flashes and other normal manifestations of perimenopause. Unwanted side effects occur with these drugs, in part, because their molecules differ in some significant ways from natural hormone molecules. Returning to the example in the last chapter, although the *R* end of the drug's *key* fits the hormone receptor well enough to have hormone-like effects, the *E* end may not fit some important enzyme locks. As a result, the drug may cause breast tenderness, gallstones, or other unpleasant symptoms.

POSSIBLE UNWANTED EFFECTS OF CONVENTIONAL "ESTROGEN" REPLACEMENT

- Breast tenderness
- Headaches
- Leg cramps
- Gallstones
- Worsened uterine fibroids and endometriosis
- Vaginal bleeding
- High blood pressure
- Blood clots
- Nausea & vomiting
- Fluid retention
- Impaired glucose tolerance
- Increased risk of endometrial cancer and breast cancer

Estriol Replacement

In the United States and Canada, "estrogen" replacement has usually been accomplished with Premarin,® with other patentable "estrogens," or with estradiol, a "natural" estrogen. Unfortunately, estradiol has also been used alone. In our bodies, estradiol is always accompanied by estrone and estriol. Even more unfortunately, estradiol is suspected of being the most pro-carcinogenic of the three! (Sometimes medical practice seems perverse, doesn't it?) Estriol is thought by many to be anti-carcinogenic (which may partly be the reason there's normally more estriol in our bodies than estradiol and estrone combined). Perhaps for this reason, many European studies on estrogen replacement have used estriol alone.

The molecular structure of replacement natural estriol is exactly the same as that of the estriol the body produces itself. The body cannot tell them apart. As a result, natural hormone replacement using natural estriol has been found to be as effective as or better than horse "estrogens" and other patentable treatments at reducing the symptoms of estrogen deficiency. Estriol stimulates the same estrogenic receptors as the others, but its effects are much more brief. Moreover, estriol produces virtually none of the common unwanted side effects of the patentable "hormones."

Clinical studies, mostly from Europe, have shown that women who use estriol replacement experience a reduction in symptoms, like hot flashes and thinning of vaginal tissue (vaginal atrophy). Exactly how estriol (and other forms of estrogen) relieve hot flashes is still unclear. Estriol appears to prevent or reverse vaginal atrophy by increasing the number of cells in the vaginal tissue, and by improving the elasticity and lubrication of this tissue.

In one major trial, 22 practicing gynecologists from 11 large hospitals in Germany treated 911 perimenopausal women with estriol and evaluated them regularly for five years. Estriol was found to be "very effective" against common menopausal symptoms and "well-tolerated" with "no significant side effects."

A Swedish study evaluated estriol treatment for up to 10 years in 40 postmenopausal women with urinary incontinence (leaky bladders). Significant improvement was seen in 30 (75%) of the women, including eight whose ability to regulate urination completely returned to normal.

In this same study, symptoms of atrophic vaginitis (vaginal dryness, painful intercourse) disappeared in 79% of the women after four months of estriol treatment. After 12 months, 98% were symptom-free.

Urinary and vaginal infections, also quite common in post-menopausal women, are often caused by the overgrowth of bacteria and yeasts that do not belong, but are able to thrive because the normal hormone balance is disrupted. Many of these infections can be prevented by estriol replacement, which appears to promote the growth of *healthy* bacteria that normally live in these areas and push out the *unhealthy* bacteria and yeasts.

Estrogen and Blood Clotting

Abnormal blood clotting due to "estrogen" has been a concern ever since the early days of the birth control pill, which contained a relatively large amount of "estrogen" and was associated with a higher risk of *thrombophlebitis* (clotting in inflamed veins, usually leg veins). Thrombophlebitis also occurs more often during pregnancy, when estrogen (primarily estriol) levels are also unusually high. Blood clots sometimes travel, lodging in the heart, lungs, and brain, often with devastating consequences.

Over the years, "estrogen" levels have been reduced in oral contraceptives, and the risk of blood clots has also diminished. In women on conventional HRT, which employs doses of "estrogen" that are generally far lower than those used in *the pill,* the risk is very small. Nevertheless, it is significantly higher than it is in women who are not on conventional hormone replacement. A recent retrospective analysis of postmenopausal women published in *The Lancet,* for example, found that women who used horse estrogen had a risk of venous thromboembolism (venous clots which travel) two to seven times higher than those who did not. Higher daily doses of "estrogen" were associated with a greater risk.

Does estriol increase the risk of thromboembolism? At high doses, such as those occurring during pregnancy, it's possible. Over the years, I've observed that combinations of cod liver oil and vitamin E help enormously in the treatment of phlebitis, and when taken regularly, are nearly 100% effective as preventive treatment, even during pregnancy.

Since natural hormone replacement produces all of the benefits without the unwanted adverse effects of the patentable "hormones" (an increased risk of cancer and abnormal blood clotting), conventional HRT is a needlessly dangerous option.

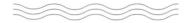

CHAPTER 5

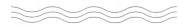

Preventing and Reversing Osteoporosis

MANY WOMEN FEAR osteoporosis when menopause approaches. Who hasn't had a grandmother chronically hunched over due to the weakening and compression of her vertebrae, or an aunt who broke her hip and died soon after?

In osteoporosis, the bones lose calcium (as well as other minerals) and become thinner, weaker, and increasingly prone to fracture, even after mild impact, or even no apparent impact. Both fall-and-fracture and first fracture, then fall are thought to be common ways for women with osteoporosis to break their hips.

The most vulnerable bones include those in the hip (femoral neck), wrist, shoulder, ribs, and spine, all of which contain relatively large amounts of sponge-like (cancellous or trabecular) bone. The longer bones of the arms and legs are much denser and stronger, and consequently, are less likely to suffer the effects of osteoporosis.

Many years of osteoporosis are responsible for the dowager's hump in some elderly women, due to the fracture and subsequent compression of vertebrae. A broken hip due to a severely weakened femoral neck too often marks the beginning of the end for many people with osteoporosis.

Osteoporosis occurs because bone, hard as it is, is a dynamic tissue that is constantly being remodeled throughout life. The remodeling process has two main phases. First, cells called *osteoclasts* travel throughout bone tissue. When they come upon older bone, they dissolve or resorb it, leaving tiny, unfilled spaces, or pores, in its place.

Following in the wake of the osteoclasts are cells called

osteoblasts, which enter these pores and begin construction of new bone tissue. Throughout youth and into middle age, bone remodeling reflects a healthy balance between these two processes.

Osteoporosis means basically that the osteoclasts are outrunning the osteoblasts, resulting in a relative loss of bone tissue. Women's bone mass reaches its peak during the early to mid-30s, after which it begins a slow decline until menopause. After menopause, bone loss accelerates considerably, often reaching a rate of 1% to 1.5% per year.

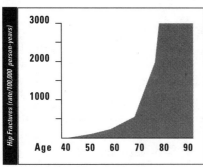

Source: Arneson, et al. Epidemiology of diaphyseal and distal fermoral fractures in Rochester, Minnesota, 1965-1984. *Clinical Orthopedics.* 1988;234:188-194

Fig. 5.1: Rate of Hip Fractures Increases After Menopause.

Both men and women develop osteoporosis, but the incidence is much higher in women after menopause. The results of surveys carried out in eight European countries show that the incidence of hip fracture doubles every five to seven years after age 45 (Fig. 5.1). A random sample of 300 women examined by the Mayo Clinic in Rochester, Minnesota, found that 18% of women age 50 or older had one or more fractured vertebrae due to osteoporosis.

Osteoporosis is a complex disease with several causes, but the fact that the process of bone loss accelerates so rapidly after menopause (or after surgical removal of the ovaries) was an early clue that estrogens and progesterone might have something to do with it. One possibility is that estrogens mediate the metabolism of vitamin D, which is needed for bone formation. More importantly, estrogens and progesterone may act directly on bone tissue to enhance mineral deposition and slow the rate of natural bone cell loss. Thus, as estrogen and progesterone levels drop, so would bone mineral density.

It makes sense that if osteoporosis were caused by an estrogen/progesterone deficiency, replacing the missing estrogen/progesterone might help prevent the loss of bone or, at least, slow its

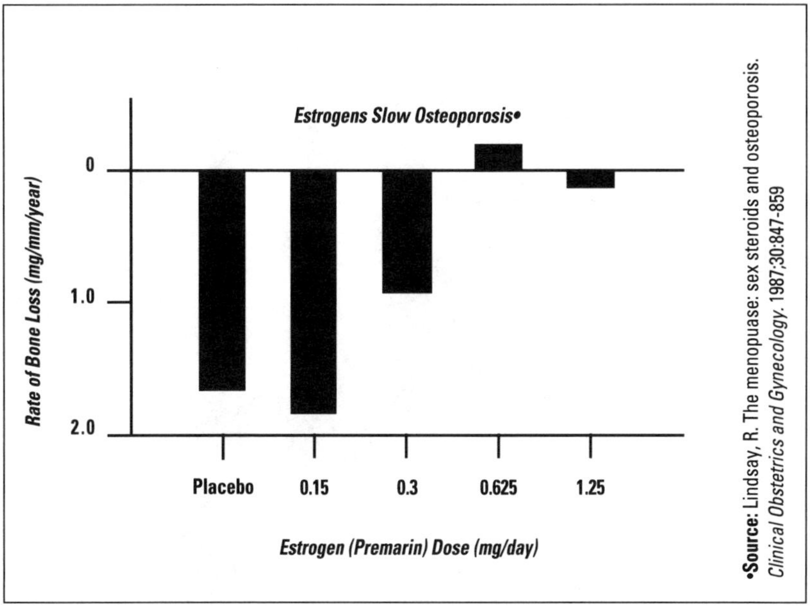
Estrogens Slow Osteoporosis•
Rate of Bone Loss (mg/mm/year)
0
1.0
2.0
Placebo
0.15
0.3
0.625
1.25
Estrogen (Premarin) Dose (mg/day)
•Source: Lindsay, R. The menopuase: sex steroids and osteoporosis.
Clinical Obstetrics and Gynecology. 1987;30:847-859

Fig. 5.2: "Estrogens" Slow Osteoporosis

progress. And that is essentially what most scientific studies have shown. Figure 5.2 shows the results of one such study demonstrating that Premarin® treatment can slow or even halt bone loss. (Unfortunately, large scale studies have only been funded for patentable "hormones.") Overall, it appears that the longer a woman uses an "estrogen" replacement, the lower her risk of hip fracture. After about ten years, the risk reduction tends to level off at about 50%. The incidence of vertebral fracture may be reduced by as much as 90% after ten years of "estrogen" replacement.

The earlier "estrogen" replacement is started, the better the result. This is illustrated in Figure 5.3, which compares bone density in three groups of women who had their ovaries surgically removed (surgical menopause) and were started on "estrogen" replacement (using horse estrogen) immediately after surgery, three years after surgery, or six years after surgery, respectively. Note that when "estrogen" was started immediately, virtually no loss in bone density occurred. When "estrogen" was started after three years, bone density was lower and then stabilized. Started

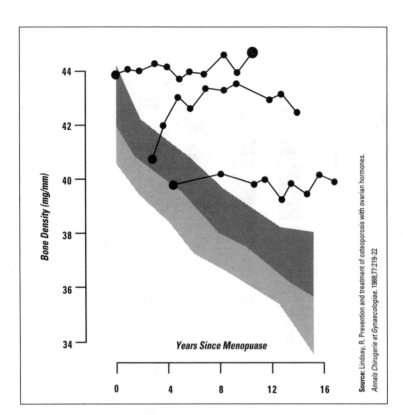

Fig. 5.3: *Estrogens Preserve Bone Density, But They Don't Restore It.*

after six years, bone density was still lower and stabilized at an even lower level. (The cross-hatched area represents the loss of bone density that would be expected if the women did not replace estrogen.)

This study also makes another very important point about "estrogen" replacement that often gets lost. Look at Figure 5.3 again. While bone loss was stabilized by "estrogen" replacement, no bone was regained. "Estrogen" replacement does not rebuild bone, it only slows loss.

So, does "estrogen" replacement alone prevent osteoporosis? In one way, we could say "Yes," since it prevents, or at least slows, the progression of osteoporosis. Most data show that "estrogen" replacement can reduce the risk of hip fractures by about 50%. Do

NATURAL HORMONE REPLACEMENT/CHAPTER FIVE

"estrogens" cure osteoporosis? Certainly not. If your bones are already weakened by the time you start taking estrogens, they're going to stay weak.

Is there anything you can do to make them stronger? Absolutely!

Natural Progesterone vs. Patentable "Progestins"

Women who take natural progesterone (and/or natural estrogens) in physiologic doses (i.e., doses that reproduce normal levels in the body), report virtually no unwanted effects. [According to John R. Lee, M.D., the Northern California physician who pioneered the study of natural progesterone in women after menopause, natural progesterone does have *one* side effect. Dr. Lee says, "That guy across the room will get better looking." He points out that progesterone is at least partly responsible for the sex drive in women. "Presumably this is Nature's way of assuring a meeting of the egg with a sperm after ovulation," states Dr. Lee.]

This is far from the case with patentable "progesterones" ("progestins" or "progestogens"). A quick look at the approved labeling for Provera® (medroxyprogesterone) reveals that more than 60% of the text is devoted to Contraindications, Warnings, Precautions, and Adverse Reactions. Provera® is a serious drug with many serious consequences, including the possibility of:

• Birth defects, if Provera® is taken when pregnant	• Impaired glucose tolerance
• Breast cancer	• Breast tenderness and milk production
• The formation of blood clots, especially in the lungs or the brain	• Skin rash
• Fluid retention, swelling	• Acne
• Breakthrough bleeding, or other menstrual irregularities	• Hair loss, or unwanted facial hair growth
	• Weight gain and depression

The Physicians' Desk Reference *(PDR)*, which contains the labeling for most prescription drugs sold in the United States, lists ten different Provera®-like drugs with "progesterone"-like actions ("progestins"). Many women who start taking these patentable "hormones" find the unwanted effects to be so unpleasant that they stop "HRT" altogether, thus giving up all its potential life-enhancing and life-extending benefits.

All these progesterone wannabes generally have the same unwanted effects, because not one of them is really progesterone. Like natural estrogens and patentable "estrogens," the chemical structures of progesterone and the patentable progestin Provera® are quite similar (Fig. 5.4). It is this similarity that enables Provera® to perform many of the functions that progesterone normally does. But the two molecules also have some important differences that account for the many unwanted effects that Provera® and similar drugs cause.

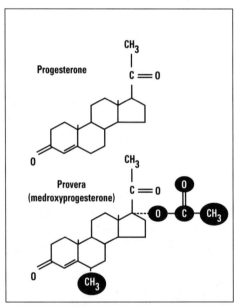

Fig. 5.4: Molecular Structure of Natural Progesterone vs. Medroxyprogesterone

What Does Real Progesterone Do?

As we discussed in Chapter 2, one of progesterone's primary roles during the menstrual cycle is to help make the uterus ready for implantation of a new embryo—the first major event after fertilization of the egg—in the nine months of human gestation. If the egg is not fertilized, progesterone production temporarily ceases, and the uterus sheds its endometrial lining.

At the same time it's helping drive the menstrual cycle, progesterone is also performing several other vital, but less well-known functions (see box). Among the most important of these are building new bone tissue and countering the tendency of estrogen to induce excess growth in the endometrial lining of the uterus. In extreme cases, excess growth can turn cancerous. Progesterone is also a major precursor for other hormones, like the estrogens and testosterone. If the progesterone spigot is turned off, as occurs at menopause, estrogen and testosterone levels may also fall.

Progesterone Builds Strong Bones

The person who has done the most to show postmenopausal women how to actually restore bone tissue is Dr. John R. Lee. Working independently and with minimal financial resources, Dr. Lee has explored the relative value of estrogens and progesterone for building bone tissue after menopause. His research points clearly in the direction of natural progesterone and raises several important questions regarding the true value of estrogens. There are several things wrong with giving

SOME OF PROGESTERONE'S MANY ROLES
• Precursor of other sex hormones (estrogen and testosterone) and cortisone
• Maintains lining of uterus
• Promotes the survival of the embryo and fetus throughout gestation
• Protects against fibrocystic breasts
• Natural diuretic
• Promotes fat burning for energy (thermogenesis)
• Acts as a natural antidepressant
• Aids thyroid hormone action
• Normalizes blood clotting
• May help maintain sex drive
• Helps keep blood sugar levels normal
• Normalizes zinc and copper levels
• Promotes proper cell oxygen levels
• Protects against endometrial cancer
• Helps protect against breast cancer
• Promotes bone building and protects against osteoporosis

estrogens all the credit for preventing osteoporosis, Dr. Lee argues:

• Since the mid-1970s, when the link between unopposed estrogen and endometrial cancer was discovered, nearly all the women who have taken patentable "estrogens" in osteoporosis studies have also taken a patentable "progestin." Why was "estrogen" given all the credit?

• "Estrogen replacement" seems to have a bone benefit for only about five years after menopause. Women who are many years past menopause would likely gain very little from starting estrogen replacement.

• Studies showing that "estrogens" slow bone loss usually

ignore bone rebuilding. As far as we know, "estrogens" (even real estrogens) do nothing to form new bone, but progesterone does.

• Osteoporosis actually begins as much as five to 20 years before menopause, when the ovaries are still functioning and estrogen levels are still high.

While replacement of all missing or deficient hormones is always best, Dr. Lee's research suggests that progesterone is more important in combating osteoporosis than are estrogens. While replacement estrogen may prevent bone loss, replacement progesterone leads to new bone formation, actively increasing bone mass and density. Taken with estrogens, progesterone can even *reverse* osteoporosis, which estrogens can't do alone.

Over a period of about ten years, Dr. Lee treated many women with hormone replacement therapy including natural progesterone. During this period, he took regular bone mineral density measurements on 63 women. About 40% used "estrogen" (Premarin®) plus natural progesterone, and the remainder used progesterone only; 62 of the women used natural progesterone for at least three years. The women also took calcium supplements and maintained a diet and lifestyle designed to minimize bone loss—no smoking, no carbonated beverages, calcium-rich foods, vitamins C, D, and beta carotene supplements. The women's average age was 65.2 years, so most were well past menopause when they began hormone replacement, and many had already experienced considerable bone loss.

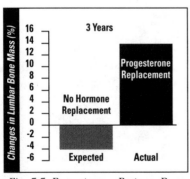

Fig. 5.5: Progesterone Restores Bone Loss in Osteoporosis

Dr. Lee found that a natural progesterone replacement cream resulted in a remarkable increase in bone mineral density. Some of his patients increased the density of their lumbar vertebrae by 20% to 25% in the first year. Over three years, the mean increase in bone density was 15.4% (Fig. 5.5). This compares quite favorably with the 4% to 5% decrease that

NATURAL HORMONE REPLACEMENT/CHAPTER FIVE

would be expected if the women had not used progesterone.

Age was not an obstacle to bone restoration. Women over age 70 had exactly the same gains as those under 70. Moreover, adding "estrogen" to the progesterone did not make any difference, somewhat supporting Dr. Lee's contention that estrogen is less important for bone health than previously thought. (Unfortunately, we don't know what would have happened if natural human estrogens had been used instead of horse estrogen.)

Virtually all the large clinical trials concerning postmenopausal bone density over the long term have employed patentable "estrogens" and "progestins." Several of these studies have actually hinted at a small bone-building benefit (3-5%). None of these results approached the dramatic improvement reported by Dr. Lee.

Results like these aren't just happening with the women with whom Dr. Lee works. Women working with other physicians have had similar results. Doris Ramirez is one. At her last visit to the Tahoma Clinic, she brought the results of her most recent bone density test, done at our local university. She looked happy as she handed them to me.

"I haven't done the calculations yet," she said, "but they're better than two years ago, and those were improved from the two years before. Here I am, 70 years old, and my bone mineral density has improved for four years in a row!"

"Congratulations! Let me do a little math," I said. "You've had slightly over 15% improvement overall. You must really be sticking to your program."

"Every bit. The diet from Dr. Gaby's book,[1] the Osteoprime® supplement that you and Dr. Gaby put together, extra calcium, and all the natural replacement hormones: triple estrogen, progesterone, DHEA, testosterone. Of course, I take a few other things, but those are the ones specifically for improving osteoporosis."

"And exercise?"

"Of course, but I'm still just doing regular walking and swimming. Remember, my bone scan four years ago showed moderate to severe osteoporosis, and you agreed that heavier exercise

---

1. Gaby, AR. *Preventing and Reversing Osteoporosis*. Keats Publishing, New Canaan, Connecticut.

might not be such a good idea."

"Right." I picked up her report, and read it again. "If you continue to improve, I might change that recommendation."

"Well, I should tell you that I've been feeling so well that I've picked it up a little already."

"No wrestling or weight lifting?"

"No, but I have gotten back on my bicycle again. I'm not nearly as afraid of falling and breaking something as I was. Of course, I'm still being careful and not trying to keep up with the grandkids."

If progesterone is so good at building bone, one might wonder why no one ever noticed before. Sadly, before Dr. Lee, no one had even bothered to look. (A cynic might say it's because progesterone isn't patentable.) "Progestins" were added to "estrogen replacement" basically from necessity—to oppose the carcinogenic potential of patentable "estrogen." Until recently, no one was really interested in the effect of "progestin" on bone metabolism. That was thought to be the job of "estrogen."

Even in 1997, in the face of positive results, conventional medicine remains blind to the bone-building role of natural progesterone. For example, consider the results of the Postmenopausal Estrogen/Progestin Interventions (PEPI) trial, a large, long-term, prospective study conducted by the National Institutes of Health (NIH) to assess the effects of "hormone replacement therapy" using Premarin® plus either Provera® or natural progesterone (taken orally) on bone and cardiovascular health.

The *PEPI* trial, published in the Journal of the American Medical Association (JAMA), showed that after three years, women receiving placebo rather than "HRT" lost an average of 2.8% of the bone mineral density in their spines and 2.2% in their hips. By contrast, those who adhered to a "standard HRT" program (Premarin® plus either Provera® or natural progesterone), gained an average of 5.1% in their spines and 2.3% in their hips. Despite these encouraging results, the headline on a press-release issued by the American Medical Association (AMA) read: "Estrogen Therapy Increases Bone Mineral Density," (italics added)—completely ignoring the role of progesterone or progestin!

The beneficial effects of natural progesterone on bone building that Dr. Lee found should really come as no surprise to medical doctors who've been paying attention to research on the role of progesterone in bone metabolism. Numerous studies of laboratory animals, tissue samples in test tubes, and women have explored how progesterone can influence bone metabolism.

In one remarkable clinical trial, scientists studying premenopausal women with normal hormone levels and regular menstrual cycling found that bone metabolism rises and falls in harmony with the level of progesterone. As progesterone levels increased each month, bone density increased slightly; as progesterone levels fell, bone density decreased slightly.

As menopause approaches, women can have occasional nonovulatory cycles in which there is no corpus luteum to produce progesterone. In the absence of progesterone during nonovulatory cycles, researchers discovered that a measurable loss in trabecular (spongy) bone mass occurred.

Progesterone After Hysterectomy?

Susan Sanders heard about natural hormone replacement from her sister and came in to talk about it. "My sister likes that Triple Estrogen better than that horse estrogen, Premarin,®" she said. After some discussion, I wrote her a prescription for Triple Estrogen, along with a progesterone prescription.

"But the doctor said I don't need progesterone," she said. "Remember, I told you I had a hysterectomy several years ago, and the doctor said the only reason for Provera® with Premarin® is to reduce the risk of endometrial cancer from Premarin,® and since I've had my uterus removed, I can't possibly get endometrial cancer anymore, so I don't need Provera,® progesterone ... you know."

The first time I heard this, I had a hard time not staring in disbelief. Now, I just sighed, "When your uterus was removed, did they remove the rest of your body?"

It was her turn to stare. "Of course not, what do you mean?"

"Progesterone affects every tissue in our bodies. There are progesterone receptors—areas on cells that receive progesterone—

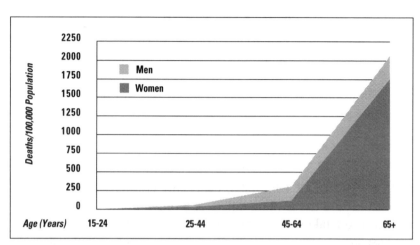

Fig. 6.2: Increasing Deaths from Heart Disease in Men and Women With Age

ease accelerates so much that by age 65, they catch up with men. Studies have shown that women who have both ovaries surgically removed in their late 30s experience a similarly rapid increase in cardiovascular death risk immediately afterward.

In addition to outright deaths, postmenopausal women have all the lesser signs of cardiovascular disease, including increases in atherosclerosis (the build-up of fatty deposits inside arteries), increases in LDL *(bad)* cholesterol and triglycerides (also *bad* in excess), and decreases in HDL *(good)* cholesterol. Taken together, these changes all spell trouble for the heart and blood vessels.

Naturally, the shutdown of the ovaries at menopause was the prime suspect in women's increase in heart disease risk. When horse estrogens like Premarin® were found to reduce the risk of heart disease, "estrogen" replacement had all the rationale it needed to become a standard therapy.

Indeed, the results of "ERT" seemed quite impressive. In one study of 1,000 women who used "estrogen" replacement for 15 years, there was a 63% reduction in expected deaths from heart disease. Another large trial followed two groups of women for 25 years. One group used "estrogen" and the other did not. The "estrogen" group had a significant decrease in the incidence of coronary artery disease, congestive heart failure, atherosclerosis,

NATURAL HORMONE REPLACEMENT/CHAPTER SIX

The beneficial effects of natural progesterone on bone building that Dr. Lee found should really come as no surprise to medical doctors who've been paying attention to research on the role of progesterone in bone metabolism. Numerous studies of laboratory animals, tissue samples in test tubes, and women have explored how progesterone can influence bone metabolism.

In one remarkable clinical trial, scientists studying premenopausal women with normal hormone levels and regular menstrual cycling found that bone metabolism rises and falls in harmony with the level of progesterone. As progesterone levels increased each month, bone density increased slightly; as progesterone levels fell, bone density decreased slightly.

As menopause approaches, women can have occasional nonovulatory cycles in which there is no corpus luteum to produce progesterone. In the absence of progesterone during nonovulatory cycles, researchers discovered that a measurable loss in trabecular (spongy) bone mass occurred.

Progesterone After Hysterectomy?

Susan Sanders heard about natural hormone replacement from her sister and came in to talk about it. "My sister likes that Triple Estrogen better than that horse estrogen, Premarin,®" she said. After some discussion, I wrote her a prescription for Triple Estrogen, along with a progesterone prescription.

"But the doctor said I don't need progesterone," she said. "Remember, I told you I had a hysterectomy several years ago, and the doctor said the only reason for Provera® with Premarin® is to reduce the risk of endometrial cancer from Premarin,® and since I've had my uterus removed, I can't possibly get endometrial cancer anymore, so I don't need Provera,® progesterone ... you know."

The first time I heard this, I had a hard time not staring in disbelief. Now, I just sighed, "When your uterus was removed, did they remove the rest of your body?"

It was her turn to stare. "Of course not, what do you mean?"

"Progesterone affects every tissue in our bodies. There are progesterone receptors—areas on cells that receive progesterone—

everywhere. Those receptors wouldn't be there without a reason. Just because the uterus is gone doesn't mean that the zillions of progesterone receptors elsewhere disappear, too! Just for one example, without progesterone, bone doesn't rebuild very well. Not taking progesterone because the uterus is gone makes as much sense as never drinking water again because one cup in a set is broken."

With what's now known about the essential role of progesterone in new bone formation, it's a shame (but not surprising) that medical gospel is still to prescribe "estrogen" only (without a patentable "progestin" or even natural progesterone) to women who have had their ovaries and uterus surgically removed prior to the time of natural menopause. Writes one author in the prestigious British medical journal, *The Lancet,* "Prevention of endometrial cancer is the only reason for adding 'progestagens' [i.e., 'progestins'] to the 'estrogen' regimen. Consequently, this strategy is unnecessary in women who have had a hysterectomy."[2]

Unfortunately, this writer is so firmly wedded to patentable "progestins" that he doesn't even consider real natural progesterone! The effect of "progestins" on bone building is, at most, minimal. They cause many unpleasant side effects and may increase the risk of heart disease (more about that later). If physicians only consider "progestins," the statement above makes sense.

Clearly, women who have had their ovaries and uterus removed (especially before the expected time of menopause) should be taking both natural estrogens and progesterone to prevent osteoporosis, as well as atherosclerosis, premature mental decline, and possibly breast cancer (see below). Progesterone has virtually none of the side effects associated with "progestins," and, as we shall soon see, it does not strip away protection against heart disease the way "progestins" do. Cancer risk or not, taking estrogen (natural or not) without progesterone, uterus or no uterus, makes no sense. There's no excuse for any of us doctors prescribing this way.

---

2. te Velde ER, van Leusden HAIM. Hormonal treatment for the climacteric: alleviation of symptoms and prevention of postmenopausal disease. *The Lancet.* 1994;343:654-658.

CHAPTER 6

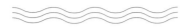

Preventing
Heart Disease

CARDIOVASCULAR DISEASES, especially coronary artery disease and stroke, are the leading killers of women in the U.S. As shown in Figure 6.1 taken from statistics for 1994 from the U.S. Centers for Disease Control and Prevention, the number of cadiovascular disease-related deaths dwarfs all other leading causes.

For many years, much more attention has been given to cardiovascular disease in men than in women. Fortunately, this is changing as it's being recognized that women have almost as much risk, just delayed by a few years. As shown by Figure 6.2, once menopause arrives, women's risk of death from heart dis-

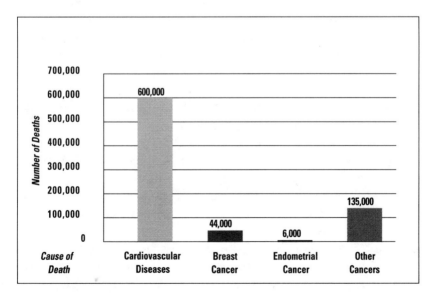

Fig. 6.1: Leading Causes of Death in Women in the United States

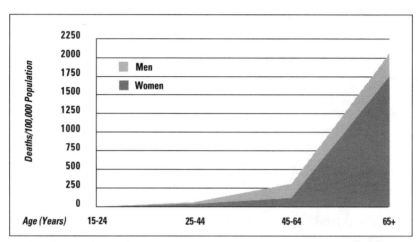

Fig. 6.2: Increasing Deaths from Heart Disease in Men and Women With Age

ease accelerates so much that by age 65, they catch up with men. Studies have shown that women who have both ovaries surgically removed in their late 30s experience a similarly rapid increase in cardiovascular death risk immediately afterward.

In addition to outright deaths, postmenopausal women have all the lesser signs of cardiovascular disease, including increases in atherosclerosis (the build-up of fatty deposits inside arteries), increases in LDL *(bad)* cholesterol and triglycerides (also *bad* in excess), and decreases in HDL *(good)* cholesterol. Taken together, these changes all spell trouble for the heart and blood vessels.

Naturally, the shutdown of the ovaries at menopause was the prime suspect in women's increase in heart disease risk. When horse estrogens like Premarin® were found to reduce the risk of heart disease, "estrogen" replacement had all the rationale it needed to become a standard therapy.

Indeed, the results of "ERT" seemed quite impressive. In one study of 1,000 women who used "estrogen" replacement for 15 years, there was a 63% reduction in expected deaths from heart disease. Another large trial followed two groups of women for 25 years. One group used "estrogen" and the other did not. The "estrogen" group had a significant decrease in the incidence of coronary artery disease, congestive heart failure, atherosclerosis, and hypertension (high blood pressure). Similar results were reported from several other large studies. The verdict seemed to be in: "estrogen" replacement protects against heart disease and stroke in postmenopausal women.

How does "estrogen" accomplish this feat? It's still a mystery, although much evidence shows that "estrogen" normalizes blood lipids. Specifically, estrogen (both patentable and natural) increases HDL cholesterol and decreases LDL cholesterol.

While these results seem clear and logical, there's still considerable controversy surrounding the value of "estrogen" for preventing heart disease. Studies designed to answer this question must be very large, costly, and carried out over many years. As a result, it's quite difficult to control all the variables that may influence the results. Unfortunately, most of the early studies were not well-controlled. There's good reason to believe that women who take "estrogen" have a generally healthier diet, exercise more, see their doctors more often, are more intelligent, earn more money, and take better care of themselves than those who do not take "estrogen." If this is so, the beneficial effects attributed to "estrogen" replacement may really be due to one or more of these other factors.

For pure research purposes, many investigators would be much happier if they could use *unopposed* "estrogen." That way, they could determine exactly what "estrogen" *alone* can do. Similarly, doctors who give "estrogen replacement" would often rather give "estrogen" alone. But, of course, that pesky cancer problem keeps popping up. As noted earlier, once it was discovered that unopposed "estrogen" increased the risk of endometrial cancer, "E"RT was forced to evolve into "H"RT. Adding a patentable "progestin" appeared to solve the problem of endometrial cancer, but it wasn't long before it was discovered that this, too, was less than a perfect solution.

"Progestin," it turned out, was eating into the protection against heart disease that "estrogen" seemed to be providing. Women on "ERT" were still faced with an unhappy choice: add "progestin" to patentable "estrogen" and receive enhanced protection against endometrial cancer, but only at the cost of reduced protection

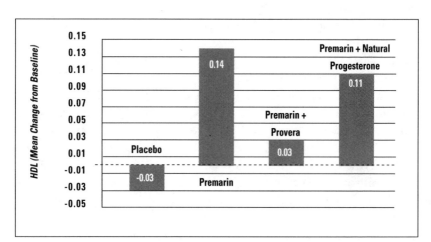

Fig. 6.3: "Estrogen" + Progesterone Keeps HDL-Cholesterol Levels High

against heart disease (not to mention a host of unwanted side effects of "progestin").

The PEPI Trial: Good News and Bad News

The most important study to examine the relative benefits and risks of various HRT regimens for heart health has been the PEPI trial, noted above with regard to osteoporosis. In this trial, 875 healthy, naturally or surgically postmenopausal women, aged 45 to 64 years, were randomly asked to take one of four "hormone" replacement programs for three years:

- Placebo
- "Estrogen" (Premarin®), unopposed
- "Estrogen" + "progestin" (Provera®)
- "Estrogen" + natural (micronized, oral) progesterone

Figure 6.3 shows the effect on HDL *(good)* cholesterol of each replacement program:

- Placebo: small decrease (0.03) in HDL
- "Estrogen" (Premarin®), unopposed: large (0.14) increase in HDL
- "Estrogen" + "progestin" (Provera®): small (0.03) increase in HDL
- "Estrogen" + natural (micronized, oral) progesterone: large (0.11) increase in HDL

NATURAL HORMONE REPLACEMENT/CHAPTER SIX

According to present knowledge, the more HDL-cholesterol, the better off the cardiovascular system is likely to be. It's obvious that "estrogen" (Premarin®) plus natural progesterone is far superior to "estrogen" (Premarin®) plus "progestin" (Provera®) for favorable effect on HDL cholesterol. [Isn't it a shame that the researchers didn't include a group of women taking natural (human) estrogen plus natural progesterone? Especially considering all the (taxpayer) money used?]

Although the researchers saw the significance as well as we can, *they buried their recommendation for natural progesterone in the very last sentence of their paper* and avoided recommending it for "women without a uterus" (osteoporosis, anyone?). They wrote: "For these women [with a uterus], 'estrogen' plus MP [micronized natural progesterone] appears to spare the endometrium and to preserve the bulk of estrogen's favorable effects on [heart disease] risk factors including HDL-C."

In an interview published by the AMA on the Internet, the PEPI trial's principal investigator, Elizabeth Barrett-Connor, MD, remarked, "If I were treating a woman primarily because she was worried about heart disease or because she had dyslipidemia [abnormal blood fats] and low HDL cholesterol, I would probably see if she wanted to take micronized progesterone. *I was quite impressed with the better effect.*" (Italics added) Then she stated, "I would like to see micronized progesterone included as a treatment in the big studies like the Women's Health Initiative." According to the president of the American Heart Association, a woman who followed Dr. Barrett-Connor's advice might reduce her risk of heart disease by 12%.

With breakthrough results this clear and as important, shouldn't we expect huge headlines urging postmenopausal women to drop everything and run out and get some natural progesterone? As our kids say, "NOT!" Somehow, this key message of the PEPI study never made it off the pages of *JAMA*. Instead, the big news was— you guessed it: "Estrogen is good for a woman's heart."

Those exact words were the first line of the *JAMA* editorial accompanying the PEPI study written by another one of the PEPI investigators, Bernadine Healy, MD, a former head of the National

Institutes of Health (NIH). What did she say about natural progesterone? Dr. Healy concluded that it needed "further study."

In the AMA Internet interview, Dr. Healy showed a bit more enthusiasm about progesterone than she did in her editorial, expressing "surprise" that it was so effective in protecting HDL and suggesting, "We have to find out more about micronized progesterone. Why is it so different from Provera®? *Physiologically, you wouldn't expect that it should be.*" (Italics added) Remember, Dr. Healy is a former head of the NIH, and yes, she really said that! She appears to really believe that Provera® and progesterone are the same thing. (Our medical schools have done a terrific job teaching the drug company line while ignoring and ridiculing natural medicine!) If nothing else, perhaps the PEPI trial will begin to open a few eyes regarding the value of natural hormones versus patentable "hormones"—not to mention why they're so different—among the leaders in the American medical community.

Actually, Dr. Healy's surprise is itself surprising. Ten years earlier, Swedish researchers published the results of a series of studies showing essentially the same thing. In these studies, published in the mid-1980s, postmenopausal women used estradiol plus either a synthetic "progestin" or natural progesterone for three to six months. Even though the duration of the Swedish studies was short (the PEPI trial has lasted more than three *years* so far), natural progesterone was found to have a generally positive effect on total and HDL-cholesterol, while the "progestin" had an overall negative effect. Unfortunately, researchers here in the United States frequently ignore, or don't even look for, similar studies done elsewhere.

The PEPI study also raised new questions about the safety of Premarin.® While it raised HDL cholesterol levels, five new cases of heart disease developed during the first three years of the study, all in the patients taking Premarin® and none in the placebo group. This suggests at least the possibility that Premarin® may actually *cause* heart disease in some postmenopausal women. Also ten women receiving Premarin® developed blood clots, four of which were serious. No women in the placebo group developed blood clots.

If *triple estrogen* or even estriol alone had been used instead of horse estrogen (Premarin®) would these problems have occurred? I suspect not, but actual studies are needed. The same question was apparently on the mind of at least two of the researchers during the AMA Internet interview. Dr. Healy raised the issue delicately, asking Dr. Barrett-Connor, "Do you have a suspicion that we haven't adequately explored what preparations we should be using in the first place? For example, some people complain that estriol was not available in our preparations yet. It's available in Europe. It's a mild estrogen, and it may have anti-breast cancer effects. It may, if anything, inhibit and certainly will not increase the risk of breast cancer."

Dr. Barrett-Connor's response was noncommittal. "Although I'm not opposed to new studies of new drugs ...," she said, and then went on to enumerate all the obstacles in the way of doing them. A cynic's translation might be: Pharmaceutical companies will freeze over before a large, well-controlled, taxpayer-financed PEPI-like trial of unpatentable estriol or *triple estrogen* ever gets done in the U.S.A.

According to the standards of modern placebo-controlled, double-blind research, there is "no evidence" that a combination of properly-timed, natural triple-estrogen and progesterone (along with DHEA and testosterone, if necessary) *will* prevent all or even part of the increase in postmenopausal cardiovascular disease. However, strictly interpreted principles of "modern science" also say there's "no evidence" to say that triple-estrogen and progesterone *won't* provide protection, either.

Simply put, "modern science" says, "We don't know, we haven't tried it." But you and all other adult women have tried this combination ... *from menarche onward!* As noted above, you have experienced the lower risk of heart and blood vessel disease that nature and creation designed them for. Any woman unfortunate enough to have her ovaries removed prior to the usual and expected age of menopause has been proven to lose this protection.

Until modern science "gets its act together" and studies the hormones we were all born with, the available evidence says very

clearly that we should continue using them, if we're to use hormone replacement at all. It's very likely that (at the very least),
they'll give us better protection against heart disease than
patentable substitutes. But it's even more likely they'll provide
protection very close to that enjoyed by all women prior to
menopause.

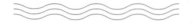

CHAPTER 7

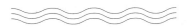

Testosterone and Other Androgens: Not Just for Men

YES, THAT TESTOSTERONE! Accused of everything from warfare and rape to Monday Night Football, the major androgenic hormone testosterone is actually vital for both men and women. And, in both men and women, testosterone levels peak during youth and decline with age. Replacing inadequate testosterone with natural testosterone can help protect the heart, improve mental alertness, make bones stronger, and revive a lagging sex life.

Although testosterone is the major androgen, some researchers consider testosterone also to be a weak estrogen. Remember (Chapter 3) that our bodies make estradiol from testosterone as well as from estrone. When estrogen levels begin to drop during perimenopause, testosterone appears to be able to pick up part of the slack. When women who have had their ovaries removed take testosterone, their levels of estrone and estradiol can rise significantly.

Cardiovascular Protection

According to evidence accumulating for decades in Europe but little known by the conventional American medical community, testosterone may play a crucial role in protecting us against atherosclerosis and heart disease. Some evidence suggests that testosterone replacement (using *natural* testosterone, of course) can reduce the risk of serious heart disease.

For more than twenty years, Dr. Jens Møller, a Danish researcher, was a leading advocate of testosterone replacement for protecting the heart. Among Dr. Møller's many important arguments is the fact that the amount of cholesterol in our diets often has little to do with the amount of cholesterol in our arteries.

Furthermore, reducing blood cholesterol with the powerful, patentable cholesterol-reducing drugs so popular with physicians in the 1990s may do more harm than good.

[Research completed after Dr. Møller's death has confirmed that patentable cholesterol-reducing drugs increase the risk of cancer and heart failure, and even increase accidents, suicide and violent death. But back to Dr. Møller's reasoning ...]

Remember, cholesterol is the basic steroid from which all other steroids in the body are derived. Cutting cholesterol levels so drastically can throw the body into a state of *negative cholesterol balance* leading to, among other disorders, impotence and impaired cardiac function showing up as angina, claudication (painful walking), and other signs of serious cardiovascular disease. "The cholesterol is wasted by going down the drain instead of building up testosterone," writes Dr. Møller. "It is totally incomprehensible to me how such a substance [an anticholesterol drug] can be used by serious practitioners in medicine, who inflict cardiovascular disease on their patients instead of curing it."

"Organisms cannot exist without cholesterol, which takes part in all cell functions," he adds. "If we interfere with this system, e.g., medically, the result may be that we decrease resistance to infection; we may even accelerate the aging process."

Testosterone Decreases Cholesterol—Safely

One of the least known secrets about natural hormones is that testosterone *decreases* cholesterol levels. In one of Dr. Møller's studies done in the late 1970s, 300 men (ages 41-82) diagnosed with cardiovascular disease received testosterone injections three times a week. The result was a reduction in circulating cholesterol in 83% of the men. (It has been my observation that natural testosterone lowers cholesterol in women as well.)

Møller points out that aging is largely a tissue breakdown *(catabolic)* process. Testosterone is a tissue building *(anabolic)* hormone; it promotes the building up of body tissues like muscle and bone. (The *anabolic steroids* some athletes take to bulk up are highly potent patentable versions of testosterone with serious side effects. Natural testosterone is safe when used properly. Sound familiar?) Evidence suggests that testosterone can slow the slide into *catabolism* (tissue breakdown) associated with aging and can help restore the body's physiologic processes to a more youthful condition.

When people with cardiovascular disease take testosterone, their circulation improves. "The claudication patient walks without difficulty; angina pectoris attacks slowly disappear; gangrene heals, and signs of hypoxia on the ECG [electrocardiogram] are normalized," states Dr. Møller.

He believes some people with serious heart disease can substitute testosterone replacement therapy for dangerous and expensive surgical procedures, such as an angioplasty or coronary artery bypass, which are often only temporarily successful at unclogging coronary arteries. Noting that people considered to be candidates for coronary artery bypass surgery often have the same types of ECG abnormalities shown to be improved by testosterone, Møller writes, "It is only natural to ask why testosterone is not tried before submitting the patient to the risks of angiography and operation."

Enhancing Libido

In both men and women, testosterone increases the desire for sexual activity. Although estrogen can also have a libido-enhancing effect, testosterone's effect is usually far greater. This may seem like startling news—testosterone making women sexier? In fact, scientists have known about this effect of testosterone for nearly half a century. In a well-controlled, double-blind, placebo-controlled study published in 1950, it was found that menopausal women receiving "testosterone" treatment (un-natural *methyltestosterone,* in this case) increased their *libidinous drive* by 65%. By comparison, those women who received "estrogen" increased by only 12%.

Other researchers who have evaluated the sexual effects of testosterone report that women receiving this hormone after menopause experience increases in:

- Sexual response
- Frequency of sexual intercourse

- Sexual desire
- Number of sexual fantasies
- Level of sexual arousal

Of course, these studies were all done with synthetic patentable forms of the hormone, but there's no reason to believe that natural testosterone would be any less effective. One thing is certain, natural testosterone is bound to be safer. While testosterone is probably not the answer to all sexual problems, it seems to work well for a large number of postmenopausal women who thought a joyful and satisfying sex life was only a distant memory of youth.

Testosterone Helps Build Strong Bones, Too

We've already discussed the vital roles estrogen and progesterone play in preventing—and even reversing—osteoporosis. Not to be overlooked here also is testosterone. Of course, it's well-known that many athletes enhance their muscle and bone strength by taking dangerous synthetic testosterone-like drugs. Exactly how testosterone works to enhance bone building is not yet understood, although some research suggests that it may increase calcium retention.

The lesson here, though, is that natural testosterone can also be effective in women for preventing and reversing osteoporosis. In women with osteoporosis, levels of estrogen, progesterone, and testosterone are all likely to be deficient. In those women who have experienced rapid bone loss, both estrogen and testosterone levels have been found to be low. A recent study has shown that women with osteoporosis who took a combination of estrogen and testosterone *increased* their bone density, an effect previously demonstrated only with progesterone.

DHEA—"Junk" Hormone No More

Until a few years ago, DHEA (dehydroepiandrosterone) was considered a *junk* hormone, an intermediate branch in the steroid family tree with no other particular significance. Today, the story is quite different. In his 1996 book *The Superhormone Promise,* which includes the most complete summary of DHEA research so far published, Dr. William Regelson called DHEA: "the superstar of superhormones."

If you look back at Figure 3.2, you can get an idea why DHEA may be so important. Note that DHEA occupies a central position in the steroid hierarchy. Produced from cholesterol by way of pregnenolone, DHEA is an androgen that is metabolized to form androstenedione, which begets testosterone which begets estradiol and then estrone, and finally, estriol.

It stands to reason that reduced DHEA levels can translate into reductions of these other hormones, particularly the other androgens, androstenedione and testosterone. And while reductions in the hormones derived from DHEA will have numerous well-documented effects on health, many of which we have already discussed, it is now becoming apparent that a low level of DHEA itself can be detrimental.

Men usually have more DHEA than women, but the rate of decline is about the same for both sexes. In men, about half the DHEA is lost by age 40, in women by age 45. By age 80, both men and women have only about 15% of their peak DHEA levels.

We are just beginning to understand the benefits that can be achieved by restoring DHEA levels to their youthful peak. Consider some of these facts regarding DHEA and health:

- Women with most types of breast cancer have been found to have abnormally low levels of DHEA.
- When laboratory rats are given an injection of DHEA prior to being exposed to a potent carcinogen, they remain cancer-free.
- DHEA protects against heart disease by lowering cholesterol and preventing blood clots.
- DHEA has been shown to improve memory.
- DHEA treatment strengthens the immune system and protects against autoimmune diseases like lupus erythematosus and rheumatoid arthritis.
- DHEA prevents bone loss.
- DHEA may promote reduction of body fat.
- Because it promotes the formation of other steroid hormones, DHEA can help alleviate menopausal symptoms and/or reduce the amount of other hormones required.

- DHEA has been reported to enhance libido, reduce impotency, and increase feelings of well-being while reducing depression and fatigue.

Not just estrogen and progesterone, but many other hormones, including testosterone, growth hormone, melatonin, and DHEA, reach their peak levels before or during the third decade of life and then begin a gradual decline of about 2% per year. Research clearly indicates that replacing inadequate levels of these important hormones can, among other positive effects, help protect the heart, improve mental alertness, make bones stronger, and revive a lagging sex life. We are just beginning to understand the health benefits that can be achieved by restoring levels of these important hormones to their youthful peak.

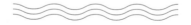

CHAPTER 8

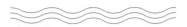

Hormone Replacement and Cancer

THE DARKEST CLOUD hanging over "hormone replacement therapy" as practiced in the United States today is cancer, especially breast cancer. The increased risk of endometrial cancer from "ERT" is largely eliminated when women take a patentable "progestin" or natural progesterone along with their "estrogen" (making it "HRT"), but the risk of breast cancer remains highly controversial.

Scores of large, sophisticated, expensive studies have been done over the years to try to answer one key question: Does replacement *horse* estrogen cause *human* breast cancer? (I'm NOT making this up! You, I, and any reasonable high school science student would want to know if replacement *human* estrogen causes *human* breast cancer. But then, you, I, and reasonable high school students don't own patents and make huge amounts of money selling horse estrogen.)

Despite all the time and money thrown at (some might say, wasted on) the problem of "HRT" and human breast cancer, the answer still remains elusive. There's no direct proof "HRT" causes breast cancer, but at the same time, it's not possible to say that it doesn't. In the face of this uncertainty, though, three facts remain indisputable:

- In nearly all the large scale studies that have examined the relationship between estrogen replacement and cancer, the "estrogens" used have been estrone + equilin (Premarin®), estradiol, or ethinyl estradiol.
- The results of many studies in laboratory animals and cell cultures have confirmed that estrone, equilin, estradiol, and

ethinyl estradiol can all cause cancer in endometrial and breast tissue.

- Some researchers think estriol has virtually no propensity to cause cancer, and that it reduces the carcinogenic activity of other estrogens and other carcinogenic chemicals in breast tissue. Others, especially those working with estriol in "unnatural" ways in experimental animals, believe estriol may have carcinogenic potential. (More about this later.)

No large studies have been done in a human population to examine the possible risk of cancer associated with estriol (or *triple estrogen*). However, a large amount of clinical and laboratory evidence dating back to the mid-1960s has been collected that addresses the issue of estriol and cancer. This research strongly suggests that estriol has less cancer-causing potential than estrone, equilin, estradiol, and ethinyl estradiol, and that estriol may actually *inhibit* the carcinogenic activity of these other "estrogens."

Nature "thinks" that estriol is important enough to constitute a majority of a woman's circulating estrogens between menarche and menopause. Modern science suggests that estriol may be a safer and more effective alternative to conventional "HRT." It's about time for researchers to examine Nature more closely and perform some very serious estriol research. (Since our bodies don't contain 100% estriol, research on a combination of all three natural estrogens in natural proportions would be even better, but serious estriol research would at least be a step in the right direction.)

How Some "Estrogens" May Cause Cancer

Like testosterone, estrogens are also growth-promoting hormones. One of estrogen's primary roles is the stimulation of growth and proliferation of cells of the endometrial lining of the uterus and cells of the breasts in preparation for pregnancy and lactation. Estrogens accomplish this by stimulating estrogen receptors located on cells at these sites.

Stimulating cell proliferation, by itself, is normally not enough to cause cancer, though. Some other event must initiate the cancer, perhaps by altering cellular DNA. According to this theory, estrogens enlarge the pool of target cells that may become cancerous. Estrogens may also promote the growth of already-established cancer. There are two primary exceptions to this, exceptions that go in dramatically opposite directions: First, the synthetic "estrogen" diethylstilbestrol (DES) may be capable of both initiating a cancer on its own and promoting its growth. Second, estriol (when used in a way that mimics Nature) is unlikely to initiate cancer.

In the endometrium, the tendency of "estrogens" to induce proliferation is opposed by progesterone (or patentable "progestins"). In breast cells, the picture is much less clear. It appears possible that "estrogen" stimulation of already cancerous breast cells is much less opposed by progesterone (or "progestins") than "estrogen"-induced stimulation of endometrial cells.

Built-In Cancer Protection

Unlike other "estrogenic" treatments, such as horse estrogens or 100% estradiol, there is no evidence that estriol at reasonable doses stimulates excessive proliferation of endometrial cells, which is a precursor to endometrial cancer. Estriol actually may antagonize the proliferative activities of other estrogens, probably because it competes for and benignly occupies estrogen receptor sites that would otherwise be occupied by the other more proliferation-oriented estrogens.[1] Thus, it appears that Nature may use estriol to partially block these powerful hormones before they can do harm.

The more benign nature of estriol is illustrated by comparing the *proliferative doses* of the various estrogens used for replacement therapy. (The *proliferative dose* is the dose that produces full endometrial cell growth, as in preparation for embryo implantation). The higher the proliferative dose, the more benign (some would say weaker) the estrogen; the lower the proliferative dose, the more potent (some would say more potentially dangerous) the estrogen.

Studies in experimental animals have shown that the proliferative dose of estriol is at least twice as high as that for horse estrogens (equilin + estrone) and estradiol, and 60 to 75 times higher than that of the synthetic estrogen ethinyl estradiol.

This means that it takes far more estriol than the other "estrogens" to cause significant cell proliferation, which caused researchers for many years to dismiss estriol as a *weak* estrogen. (No one thought to ask if *weaker* might not sometimes be better.) This translates into a reduced or even negligible risk of endometrial cancer from estriol.

Even the characterization of estriol as a weak estrogen has been proven to be mistaken in some circumstances. While it's certainly less potent in causing proliferation, it is adequately potent in performing other important estrogenic functions. "It is remarkable," one German researcher wrote, "that it [estriol] does not proliferate the endometrium when given one dose a day." He strongly recommended estriol for women with menopausal complaints, calling it "an effective and safe hormone preparation."[2]

By contrast, since 1982, many women have told me that it takes more milligrams of estriol (by itself) than of triple *estrogen* to "handle menopausal symptoms." A very few women say that estriol by itself in any dose "just isn't enough" and that estradiol and estrone (the other two natural estrogens) must be added in natural proportions to "get the job done." For this reason, *triple estrogen* may be the better choice.

If Henry Lemon, MD, is correct, estriol may be Nature's own built-in cancer protection. During the 1960s and 1970s, Dr. Lemon, a long-time physician, medical researcher, and former head of the division of gynecologic oncology at the University of Nebraska College of Medicine, studied the apparent ability of estriol to protect women against breast cancer.

Dr. Lemon first got interested in estriol because this estrogen appeared to have the ability to compete with estrone and estradiol for estrogen receptor sites. With estriol occupying estrogen receptor sites, estrone and estradiol (both known to be slightly carcinogenic) are crowded out, so there's less opportunity for them to stimulate endometrial and breast cell proliferation.

Work published prior to Dr. Lemon's had already demonstrated that estradiol and estrone were both capable of promoting abnormal cell proliferation, including endometrial and breast cancer. It was also well-known that the body treats these two hormones with extreme care, converting them to estriol rapidly and irreversibly. Estriol, however, had no carcinogenic tendencies, as far as anyone knew.[3]

"Was it possible," asked Dr. Lemon, "that some women who develop breast cancer have too little estriol relative to estradiol and estrone circulating in their bodies?" While there had long been suspicion that estrogen was somehow related to breast cancer, until Dr. Lemon came along, no one had thought to look at the levels of each of the three primary estrogens separately to see how each one related to cancer.

To answer his question, Dr. Lemon ran a preliminary study in which he employed a urinary estrogen quotient *(Eq)*, which was simply a measure of the ratio of estriol to the total of estradiol + estrone in the urine over a 24-hour period; the higher the quotient, the more estriol there is relative to estradiol and estrone.[4]

In 34 women with no signs of breast cancer, Dr. Lemon found the *Eq* to be a median of 1.3 before meno-

$$\frac{\text{Estriol } (\mu g/24 \text{ hr})}{\text{Estradiol} + \text{Estrone } (\mu g/24 \text{ hr})} = Eq$$

pause and 1.2 afterward, with only 21% of the women below 1.0 (less estriol than estrone plus estradiol). The picture was quite different in the 26 women with breast cancer. Their median *Eq* was 0.5 before menopause and 0.8 afterward, with 62% below 1.0 (Fig 8.1). Thus, the women with breast cancer seemed to be making substantially less estriol relative to the other estrogens than women without breast cancer.

Dr. Lemon's results raised more questions. Does this apparent hormone imbalance open the door to breast cancer? Is it a reliable biologic marker of breast cancer risk? Could it be used to predict which women were vulnerable to the disease but had not yet developed it? And most importantly, could restoring the natural hormone balance prevent breast cancer and perhaps even treat ongoing disease? These are intriguing questions that still need good solid scientific answers.

Some researchers have published work disputing Dr. Lemon's findings, while others have published research supporting him.

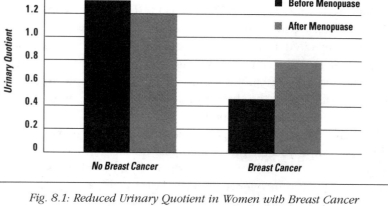

Fig. 8.1: Reduced Urinary Quotient in Women with Breast Cancer

The issue is complicated by the fact that a woman's level of estriol when breast cancer becomes apparent may not be as important as a deviation from the norm in her estriol levels as a young woman.

One supportive article in the *New England Journal of Medicine* looked at the estriol question from a different point of view. The researchers found the levels of estrone and estradiol (the known procarcinogenic estrogens) in the blood of 150 sisters and daughters of women with breast cancer to be significantly higher than in a matched control group. They also found blood levels of estrone and estradiol to be higher in 36 teenage daughters of women with breast cancer. They noted studies showing that American women (who, as a group, have higher rates of breast cancer) have lower levels of estriol than Asian women (who, as a group, have lower levels of breast cancer), especially at the time the studies were done. The researchers pointed out that Asian women in Hawaii—whose breast cancer levels were midway between those of Asian women in Asia and American women—also had levels of estriol midway between American women and Asian women in Asia. Clearly, much more research, including

NATURAL HORMONE REPLACEMENT/CHAPTER EIGHT

ESTRIOL CAUSES CANCER IN MICE ... OR DOES IT?

A 1989 STUDY CONDUCTED in Japan demonstrates just how difficult it is to draw conclusions about the link between hormones and cancer. The researchers first injected mice under the skin with cancer cells (a type of lymphoma, cancer of the lymph glands, that did not have estrogen receptors.) Immediately afterward, they injected the mice with one of several doses of estriol ranging from very low (1 μg) to very high (10 mg).

The growth of the cancer cells was found to be enhanced in the animals receiving estriol, most markedly in those receiving a dose of 1 mg. Does this mean estriol caused the cancer cells to grow? On first glance, one might assume this, but these researchers took a closer look and came to a very different conclusion.

They found that within three to five days of the estriol administration, the mice had levels of hyaluronic acid in their skin that were about three times higher than normal. Ordinarily, such an increase in hyaluronic acid might be seen in a positive light, since the body uses this naturally produced substance for keeping skin soft and flexible. It is also the primary lubricant in joints like the knee and hip.

The Japanese researchers wondered whether it was actually the hyaluronic acid that was helping the cancer cells grow. To test this hypothesis, they injected the same cancer cells into another group of mice, but instead of giving these mice estriol, they gave them hyaluronic acid. You can guess what happened. The cancer cells grew just as they had after the estriol.

Their conclusion: it was the excess hyaluronic acid, *not the estriol,* that was promoting the cancer. Is it possible, though, that excess estriol might promote lymphona indirectly by increasing hyaluronic acid? No, because lymph glands are not found in the skin, where hyaluronic acid is typically located. Thus, whether they were normal or cancerous, they would never be exposed to high levels of hyaluronic acid.*

---

* Kawatsu R, Ezaki T, Kotani M, Akagi M. Growth-promoting effect of oestriol in a lymphoma lacking estrogen receptors. *Br J Cancer.* 1989;59:563-568.

large-scale, long-term human trials will be necessary to answer the many unanswered questions regarding estriol's role in cancer.

Despite the absence of these large expensive clinical trials, much of the evidence that is already available is encouraging. Dr. Lemon's preliminary results make sense in the light of several findings reported by other researchers, as well as by Lemon himself:

- Laboratory animal studies totaling more than 500 rat-years have demonstrated that estriol is the most active protective estrogen ever tested against cancers of the breast induced by several potent carcinogenic agents,[5] including radiation.[6]

- Few animal studies have shown estriol to have any significant carcinogenic activity—unlike estrone and equilin, estradiol, ethinyl estradiol, DES, and other patentable "estrogens," which are routinely found to be carcinogenic. Estriol, given in high doses, given continuously (every day), or implanted under animals' skins in pellets has been found to be carcinogenic. However, when estriol is given in pulses, or in non-continuous doses (which approximates the natural pattern of estrogen secretion), it was much less or not at all carcinogenic.

- When estriol is given to rats and mice combined with estradiol and estrone, it inhibits the ability of these other estrogens to stimulate uterine growth.[7]

- Estriol gives the immune system a boost by enhancing the activity of certain cells known as phagocytes whose job it is to consume foreign invaders, such as bacteria and viruses, and cancer cells.

- In a group of premenopausal women with noncancerous breast diseases, including fibroadenoma, sclerosing adenosis, and intraductal hyperplasia, estriol excretion was found to be subnormal in 60%.[8]

- Dr. Lemon observed low estriol secretion in three women who had not yet developed cancer but had precancerous changes of the breast.[9]

- During pregnancy, a woman's body increases its secretion of estriol by 1,000 fold. After pregnancy, estriol levels drop but usually remain higher than they were prior to pregnancy. This may help explain why women who have never given birth have a higher risk of breast cancer than women who have borne a child.[10]

- On balance, the evidence arising from modern scientific research favors estriol (when used in physiologic doses according to natural timing patterns) as a noncarcinogenic, anti-carcinogenic, or at worst, lowest risk estrogenic substance. When modern science isn't crystal clear, it's always safest to mimic Nature as closely as possible. This is why NHR employs the three human estrogens in exactly the patterns established in women's bodies over tens of thousands of generations. This is undoubtedly safer than using horse hormones, other patentable estrogens, or wrongly dosed, or poorly timed or even incomplete natural estrogens, such as estradiol.

Progesterone and Breast Cancer

Unlike synthetic "progestins," which have an uncertain influence on breast cancer, two important studies employing natural progesterone have demonstrated a clear protective benefit. In one publication, researchers at the Johns Hopkins University Medical School reported on more than 1,000 women being treated for infertility who were followed for more than 20 years. The women were divided into two groups, those whose infertility was caused by a deficiency in progesterone and those whose progesterone level was normal. With all other possible influences accounted for, the women who were progesterone-deficient had a *5.4-fold greater risk of premenopausal breast cancer* compared with the women whose progesterone was normal. Even more startling was the finding that the progesterone-deficient women had a *10-fold higher rate of death from cancers of all kinds.*[11]

[Like many studies, this one contained a paradox. In menopausal women, progesterone *deficiency* was associated with a *decrease* in breast cancer. Although the decrease was not statistically significant, it's a bit of a puzzle, because *added* (not subtracted or deficient) progesterone (or "progestin") added to "ERT" is thought to generally protect against cancer. The study involved only checking progesterone levels, *not* adding supplemental progesterone, or "estrogen" or other "ERT." Perhaps these would make a difference in the outcome. As medical studies almost always say, "Further study is needed."]

The other study, conducted in Taiwan, focused on the proliferation of breast epithelial cells removed from women who had undergone a lumpectomy for breast cancer. About ten to 13 days prior to their surgery, the women were randomly assigned to apply a topical gel containing either estradiol, progesterone, estradiol + progesterone, or a placebo each day. When the researchers examined postsurgical breast tissue from around the lump, they found increased proliferation of breast epithelial cells in the samples from the women who had used the estradiol-only gel compared with placebo. By contrast, cell proliferation was significantly reduced in the tissue samples from the women who had used either the estradiol/progesterone gel or the progesterone-only gel.[12]

What About Ovarian Cancer?

The risk of developing ovarian cancer as a result of "hormone" replacement has not been investigated nearly as intensively as breast or endometrial cancer. It should be. A large, prospective study recently conducted by the Emory University School of Public Health in Atlanta, Georgia, reported about more than 240,000 peri- and postmenopausal women studied for seven years. The results indicate a significant risk associated with "estrogen" replacement. During the course of the study, 436 of the women died from ovarian cancer, and their risk of dying increased significantly with the length of time they had been taking "estrogen" replacement. Women who had used "estrogen" for six or more years but had stopped using it were found to be just as much at risk as current users.[13]

Let's Remember ...
and Research the "Forgotten Estrogen"

In a 1978 editorial in the *Journal of the American Medical Association* entitled, "Estriol, the Forgotten Estrogen?" Alvin H.

Follingstad, MD, bemoaned the lack of large clinical trials on estriol that would earn it an FDA stamp of "approval." "Do we as clinicians have to wait the years necessary for the completion of these trials before estriol becomes available to us?" he asked. "I think not. Enough presumptive and scientific evidence has been accumulated that we may say that orally administered estriol is safer than estrone and estradiol."

Two decades later, we are still waiting for those clinical trials, and what Dr. Follingstad said then is even more true today. There's nothing to be gained by waiting. If a woman is concerned about her risk of cancer from "estrogen" replacement (and who isn't?), then the logical choice (considering both modern scientific research and hundreds of thousands of years of human experience with producing and metabolizing estrogens) is estrogen containing a majority of estriol, or in some cases, estriol alone.

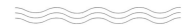

1. Hisaw FI, Velardo JT, Goolsby CM. Interactions of estrogens on uterine growth. *J Clin Endocr.* 1954;14:1134-1143.

2. Lauritzen C. Results of a 5-year prospective study of estriol succinate treatment in patients with climacteric complaints. *Hormone Metabolism Res.* 1987;19:579-584.

3. Hamilton, TH. Control of estrogen of genetic transcription and translation. *Science.* 1968; 161:649-661.

4. Lemon, HM, Wotiz, HH, Parsons, L, Mozden, PJ. Reduced estriol excretion in patients with breast cancer prior to endocrine therapy. *JAMA.* 1966;196:112-120.

5. Lemon, HM. Oestriol and prevention of breast cancer. *The Lancet.* March 10, 1973:546-547.

6. Lemon, HM. Heidel JW, Rodriquez-Sierra JF. Principles of breast cancer prevention. 1991: Paper presented at Annual Meeting of the AACR.

7. Hisaw FI, Velardo JT, Goolsby CM. Interactions of estrogens on uterine growth. *J Clin Endocr.* 1954;14:1134-1143.

8. Bacigalupo G, Schubert K. Untersuchungen uber die oestrogen auscheidung im urin bei mastopathie. *Klin Woschr.* 1960;38:804-805.

9. Lemon, HM, Wotiz, HH, Parsons, L, Mozden, PJ. Reduced estriol excretion in patients with breast cancer prior to endocrine therapy. *JAMA.* 1966;196:112-120.

10. Siitteri PK, MacDonald PC. The utilization of circulating dehydroepiandrosterone and fate for estrogen synthesis during human pregnancy. 1963;2:713-730.

11. Cowan LD, Gordis JA, Tonascia JA, Jones GS. Breast cancer incidence in women with a history of progesterone deficiency. *J Epidemiol.* 1981;114:209-217.

12. Chang KJ. Influences of percutaneous administration of estradiol and progesterone on human breast epithelial cell cycle in vivo. *Fertil Steril.* 1995;63:785-791.

13. Rodriguez C, Calle EE, Coates RJ, Miracle-McMahill HL, Thun MJ, Heath CW. Estrogen replacement therapy and fatal ovarian cancer. *Am J Epidemiol.* 1995;141:828-835.

CHAPTER 9

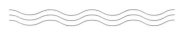

Estrogen and Senility

ONE OF THE MOST EXCITING developments in "HRT" in recent years has been the discovery of a link between low estrogen and loss of mental function, such as that which occurs in Alzheimer's disease and other forms of *senile dementia* (loss of mental function as we grow older). The biochemical mechanisms involved aren't really understood, but it is thought that estrogen somehow helps preserve and regenerate nerve cells in the brain and maintain the brain's blood supply.

Regardless of the mechanisms, though, it now appears certain that low estrogen levels don't cause Alzheimer's disease, but may be an important contributor to its progression. Preliminary data suggest that women who have not yet developed symptoms of Alzheimer's may be able to delay its onset or prevent it completely by increasing their estrogen levels. Estrogen may also prove beneficial for women who already have symptoms.

Even though Alzheimer's symptoms usually don't show up within the first 20 years after menopause, it is important not to wait until they do before beginning estrogen replacement. This is because Alzheimer's does not usually become apparent until significant brain damage has already occurred. By the third decade after menopause, 50% of women destined for Alzheimer's already have measurable brain damage, and about 50% of these will not yet have manifested any symptoms.

In a long-term Columbia University study of aging and health, more than 1,100 postmenopausal women had no signs of Alzheimer's disease at the start of the study. Those who were taking "estrogen" began to show signs of Alzheimer's at a significantly later age than those who were not on "estrogen" replacement. Furthermore, the "estrogen"-treated women had only a 5.8% risk of developing the disease compared with a 16.3% risk for the non-"estrogen"-treated women. According to the results of another study conducted at the retirement community, Leisure World, the longer women took "estrogen," the lower was their risk of developing Alzheimer's.

Even if Alzheimer's disease has already begun to affect a woman's mental function, it may not be too late to start "estrogen" (or better, natural estrogen) therapy. Several trials have found that some elderly women with senile dementia experience improved mental and emotional function with "estrogen" replacement. In one recent preliminary trial, 12 women diagnosed with Alzheimer's received either "estrogen" (estradiol via a patch) or placebo. After eight weeks, neurological tests showed that the estradiol-treated women had better memories, were more attentive, and were able to concentrate better. As soon as they stopped using the estradiol patch, these benefits diminished.

It's possible that estrogen might enhance a woman's mental ability after menopause even if she doesn't have Alzheimer's or some other form of senile dementia. In one recent study, 36 intellectually normal postmenopausal women took a battery of standard tests of mental ability before and after starting "estrogen" replacement. "Estrogen" treatment resulted in a "clear and significant" improvement in the women's mental abilities, including memory, eye-hand coordination, reflexes, and the ability to learn new information and apply it to a problem. Although it was not clear whether such laboratory improvements would translate to everyday mental functioning, these are certainly promising results.

Although we still don't understand exactly how estrogen works its beneficial effects on brain function, the growing number of studies attesting to the value of estrogen replacement in maintaining mental agility after menopause adds yet another reason to consider natural hormone replacement.

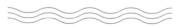

CHAPTER 10

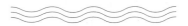

Using Natural Hormones

"IT'S TIME TO GET OFF this Premarin® and Provera® and on to natural hormones," Ingrid Johanssen said. "Harold here," she indicated her husband, "and I just found out I've been swallowing horse urine concentrate every day! And then I read something about a Dr. John Lee and natural progesterone. Apparently Provera® is about as close to real progesterone as fool's gold is to real gold!

"Well, I decided it was time to stop being a fool, so I did some investigating on my own," she continued. "I read one of your magazine articles that said we women have three basic estrogens in our bodies—*estrone, estradiol,* and *estriol,* I think—for all the years we're having menstrual cycles. And then we have progesterone, too. So the minute I read that, it made absolutely good sense to me that if I'm going to use hormone replacement, I should use *hormone* replacement, not substitution with some drug that doesn't belong in my body anyway! Also, I want to know more about DHEA and testosterone. Apparently they're replacement hormones, too, and no doctor ever mentioned them to me!"

"How long have you been taking Premarin® and Provera®?" I asked.

"Over 15 years. Started when I was 48; I'm almost 64 now. From what I've read, the risk of breast cancer is significantly greater after 15 years or so of Premarin.®"

"Likely so."

"I still can't believe it. You know, the other day we were driving by a high school, and Harold suddenly got an idea. We couldn't stop laughing, Harold had to pull off the road." She turned to her husband. "You tell the doctor, Harold."

"It's just good logic," he said. "Ingrid had just told me about the horse urine concentrate. I thought why not use the real thing? All it would take is a little re-plumbing and processing at the local high school—you know, the women's restroom—and use *human* urine concentrate instead of horse urine concentrate. Lots of hormones at all the high schools. Could be a real money-maker! Solve the school funding crisis and all that."

"Good idea. It certainly makes more sense to use human hormone concentrate in humans rather than horse hormone concentrate. Actually, that very thing was done centuries ago in China. Appears to have worked, too. As you probably know, today's natural hormone replacement uses molecules identical in every respect to human hormones, even though they're chemically changed from the starting material."

"The starting material is from *Dioscorea* yams, isn't it?"

"You *have* been doing your reading."

Harold laughed, "Once Ingrid gets going on something, she has to know everything about it."

"When it involves staying healthy, that's a very good idea," I said.

"Are you going to run hormone tests on me?"

"Yes, but not right away. We can safely assume that your own body's estrogens and progesterone are low, so we don't need to check them right away. You can start with conservative doses of estrogens, progesterone, and DHEA. After a few weeks, please have the test done and we'll readjust doses as indicated, and perhaps add testosterone. Of course, we'll pay as much attention to how you feel as to the results of the lab test."

"In all the time I took Premarin® and Provera,® no one ever ran a single test on me. How did they know whether I was on the right dose?"

I shrugged. "Who can say what a 'normal' amount of horse hormone is in a human body? Or any other patentable molecule?"

Harold laughed, "Just like testing a dog for feathers. It won't fly."

"Should I go get a blood test?" Ingrid asked.

"No, not a blood test. Even though it's less convenient, please collect a *24-hour urine specimen.* This type of test is most accurate for steroid hormones. The laboratory I work with will check the levels of all the sex hormones—all three estrogens, plus progesterone, testosterone, and DHEA—for $129. And later, when we want to check DHEA metabolites and testosterone more closely, they do that, too."

"DHEA metabo-whats? Are those even more hormones to take?"

"No. DHEA is an important hormone *on its own,* but it also metabolizes—turns into—other steroid hormones quite rapidly. If we just measured *before and after* DHEA levels, we could be seriously misled about the amount of DHEA that would be most appropriate for you. The metabolites—they're called *androsterone* and *etiocholanolone*—are measured along with DHEA to help us to make sure that too much DHEA isn't disappearing—being metabolized into—other steroid molecules. If the levels of these metabolites go too high, there quite possibly would be unwanted effects or even damage in the long run."

"And you're saying we might miss that if just DHEA were measured."

"Right."

"Told you she was a tiger on this stuff, Doc," Harold said.

"Also, some women metabolize DHEA into testosterone very efficiently, and some don't. So we start with DHEA by itself first, do the follow up testing, and then add in testosterone if the levels are still too low."

"One step at a time. Makes sense. So you'll write me prescriptions for estrogen pills?"

"We could use pills, but more and more women are using *transdermal penetrating creams* that they can rub into hormone-sensitive areas. Hormones may work a little better that way because they pass through the circulation at least once before the breakdown process starts in the liver. When we swallow anything, the liver is always the first stop, and some is broken down before it even gets used."

"And if I rub them into ... say ..."

"Places I don't have," Harold broke in.

"Right," I said. "And as an added benefit, some women have told me that after a few months of rubbing the hormone cream into the right areas, their *leaky bladder* problems cleared up."

"Well, I'm certainly glad I don't have that problem, but some of my friends do. I'll pass that along."

"And she will, too," Harold said.

So, you'll write me prescriptions for the estrogen—I guess it's called *triple estrogen*—rub-in cream, progesterone the same way, and DHEA. Later, I'll have the follow-up testing done, maybe adjust my doses, make sure both DHEA and its metabolites are all within normal, and see if I need to add testosterone or not."

"Exactly right."

"Told you, Doc."

Ingrid turned to Harold. "It's important, and I want to get it exactly right, dear. By the way, did I mention that you have an appointment next week to talk about hormone replacement for men?"

It's Simple—Just Copy Nature!

It's been repeated over and over (hope you're not getting tired of it), but it's important: unless modern science proves a point about health care with crystal clarity and beyond a doubt, it's always safest—and usually most effective—*to observe and copy Nature* in matters of health. So, if hormones are to be replaced, use *triple estrogen,* progesterone, DHEA, and (if indicated) testosterone. Please do not allow substitutions!

The *natural pattern* of circulating estrogens is:*
- 10-20% estrone
- 10-20% estradiol
- 60-80% estriol.

Like most doctors, I prefer to stay on the conservative side when prescribing. Since estriol is the least risky of the three, in 1982, I decided to routinely prescribe *triple estrogen:* 10% estrone, 10% estradiol, and 80% estriol. All compounding pharmacies carry *triple estrogen* in these proportions. The average dose is 2.5 mg. Since women's bodies always make and contain all three estro-

---

See page 127 for new data on this.

gens, I always recommend *triple estrogen* unless a woman has had cancer (see below).

Occasionally the routine prescription (10%-10%-80%) isn't strong enough even at higher doses, and perimenopausal or menopausal symptoms persist. When this happens, I first increase the total dose. If this isn't helpful I then increase the proportion of estradiol (the strongest estrogen) to 20 or 25%. If necessary, any doctor can ask the compounding pharmacist to change the proportions of each estrogen to best suit any individual (try that with Premarin®!).

Progesterone should always be prescribed along with triple estrogen. (That's what Nature does, right?). Quantities vary from 25-30 mg (after the menopause) up to 50-100mg (during the menopause) (timed as noted below), depending on each woman's age and response. Progesterone creams are available in over-the-counter form in many pharmacies and natural food stores, mostly as components of cosmetic creams. Accurate dosing is often a problem with these preparations, although this situation appears to be improving slowly.

As everyone knows, DHEA is now also available over the counter in pharmacies, natural food stores, and by mail order. I still write prescriptions for DHEA because I have a greater trust in the *USP* standard material available through compounding pharmacists. In many cases, the prices are comparable, anyway.

Over the years, I've found that *average* DHEA quantities for women range from 10 to 30 mg daily, and for men from 15 to 50 mg daily. However, follow-up testing tells me for sure, so recommendations are often adjusted higher or lower accordingly.

If testing shows that a woman's DHEA doesn't metabolize through to sufficient testosterone, she can take testosterone, too (5-10 mg daily is an average quantity). Once again, follow-up testing is mandatory to keep levels from getting neither too high nor too low, but just right.

As is the case with natural estrogens and patentable "estrogens," natural testosterone (in the right amounts at the right time) is safe. Patentable "testosterones," sometimes called *anabolic steroids,* can be very dangerous and are sometimes even illegal. Moreover, the body does not have the enzymes to convert patentable "testosterones" like *methyltestosterone* to *estradiol,* as it does with natural testosterone. Patentable "testosterones" have absolutely no place in hormone replacement therapy—for women or for men.

Cycling Replacement Hormones Nature's Way

"My doctor told me to take Premarin® and Provera® on weekdays and not on weekends."

"I just take Premarin® every day, no pauses."

"I've used the "estrogen patch" every few days for the last year or more."

We all know that Nature works in cycles. Ovaries don't secrete estrogens, progesterone, and testosterone on weekdays and not on weekends; ovaries don't secrete hormones continuously for months and years without pause. Every woman knows her sex hormones go in cycles. (By contrast, DHEA is an adrenal hormone and is secreted every day.)

"But my doctor says my uterus is gone, so cycling hormones isn't important any more."

A woman's sex hormones are not only *sent* from the ovaries in a cyclic pattern, they are also *received* in the same cyclic pattern. After approximately 40 years of *receiving cycles,* it is very likely that hormone receptors have become quite accustomed to this pattern. If this *hormone receptor timing pattern* is disrupted, especially over a period of time, it's highly likely something will go wrong, or at the very least, not function as well as it should.

Surprisingly, there's been no large research project to answer

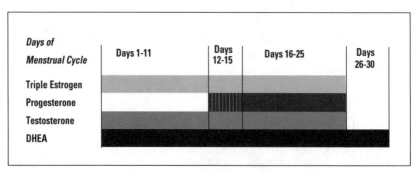

Fig. 10.1: Days of Menstrual Cycle

this important question! We might imagine that if pharmaceutical companies want to sell millions of women "estrogens" for 30 to 40 years apiece, they might fund research to determine the best timing of these hormones.

But, since this hasn't happened—and isn't likely to happen—it's best to fall back on Nature's plan. Figure 10.1 shows the pattern I usually recommend. Remember, it's not my plan, but the pattern set for us by Nature.

"What If I've Had Cancer?"

Opinions vary widely about the need for and safety of prescribing estrogens for a woman who's had cancer, especially breast, uterine, or ovarian cancer. The safest course might be avoiding estrogens of all sorts, "patentable" and natural, but for some women, heart and blood vessel disease or osteoporosis are a serious threat without hormone replacement.

When a woman's had cancer, and hormone replacement is clearly indicated, some natural medicine doctors prefer to recommend progesterone only, because it's clearly anti-carcinogenic. Others will recommend estriol (but *not* estrone or estradiol) and progesterone. DHEA is very frequently recommended because it's almost always anti-carcinogenic.

There's presently no average pattern to be followed when a woman's had cancer. But one thing is quite clear: if hormone replacement is to be used at all, *natural hormones are intrinsically safer than the patentable or incomplete versions.*

Please Work With a Doctor

Natural hormone replacement can be tricky; hormones are powerful molecules that affect our entire bodies. More is being learned about natural hormone replacement at a rapid pace, driven in part by the aging of the *baby-boom* generation. This means we have more aging doctors and researchers than ever before, too!

Melatonin is as much a craze as is DHEA; human growth hormone is here, too, needing only a drop in price to turn it into the biggest hormone replacement story ever.

As you've read, even the majority of doctors haven't studied enough to realize the importance of natural hormone replacement

(NHR) rather than conventional hormone replacement therapy (HRT). The *Resources* chapter contains information about finding a physician skilled and knowledgeable in NHR. Before you use hormone replacement of any kind, please find and work with one of these physicians.

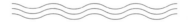

CHAPTER 11

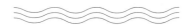

Natural Hormones From
Food and Herbs

IT'S WELL-KNOWN THAT women who live in Asian countries, such as China and Japan, have a far lower rate of death from breast cancer than women who live in the West. Moreover, when Asian women move to the U.S., Canada, or Europe, their risk of breast cancer soon rises. The same is true of menopausal symptoms, like hot flashes, insomnia, depression, and vaginal dryness, which tend to be far less common and milder in Asian women than those commonly experienced by Western women—until they move here.

What's going on here? Is it genetic? Is there something in the air? The water? The power of suggestion? Probably not. In all likelihood, the answer lies in the diet. Unlike Western women, Asian women tend to eat a lot of soy products: tofu (soybean curd), tempeh (soybean cakes), miso (soy paste), and others. When they move here, however, the amount of soy in their diets generally drops as they adapt to local customs. Could soy be a crucial dietary factor?

Soy products are known to contain large amounts of substances known as *phytoestrogens* (literally, plant estrogens). When ingested, phytoestrogens appear to function much like natural estrogens in many ways. Studies indicate, for example, that phytoestrogens increase cell growth in vaginal walls in postmenopausal women, raise HDL (the *good*) cholesterol, and reduce the risk of heart disease and osteoporosis, all without increasing the risk of cancer.

In fact, evidence suggests that phytoestrogens may actually decrease the risk of breast and endometrial cancer. Exactly how this occurs is just beginning to be understood. It is thought, for example, that phytoestrogens may block access to estrogen receptors by such procarcinogenic estrogens as estradiol. (This is the same way the natural estrogen, *estriol* and the new anti-breast cancer drug, *tamoxifen* are believed to work.) Soy products are also known to contain a variety of cancer-fighting *phytochemicals* called *isoflavonoids* and *flavonoids*. The most closely studied of these currently is *genistein,* which has been shown in a variety of animal studies to significantly retard the growth of breast cancer.

According to one estimate, about two ounces of soy products per day may be sufficient to ward off hot flashes and other symptoms and perhaps even protect against cancer and heart disease. If adding soy products to the diet is possible, then a reduction in menopause symptoms may follow, although it doesn't work for everyone.

Another potential source of phytoestrogens is the ancient grain *flax,* also known as *linseed*. Flax contains substances called *lignans,* which have been shown to have estrogen-like qualities. Like soy, flax may contain a number of phytochemicals with potent anti-cancer activity. Among the hundreds of other foods containing phytoestrogens (usually in very, very small quantities) are oats, carrots, cherry, wheat, rye, corn, chick peas, barley, hops, alfalfa, and sesame.

A very few foods have extremely small amounts of *identical-to-human* hormones. These quantities have not yet been found to be significant enough to affect human health (except possibly in the case of pomegranate, an ancient symbol of fertility). These foods include:

- Rice, apples, date palm, pomegranate – *estrone*
- French bean seedlings – *estradiol*
- Rice, licorice – *estriol*

Can Phytoestrogens Replace Natural Hormones?

Throughout this book, natural hormone replacement has been carefully defined as replacement of *natural hormones,* using molecules that are identical in every way to the ones which decline so abruptly at menopause. Phytoestrogens, by contrast, are *plant* varieties of estrogens, farther away from human estrogens in terms

BEWARE OF THE "YAM SCAM"

ALL THE NATURAL HORMONES discussed in this book (not to mention patentable "hormones") are derived from a plant as well. This plant is the Mexican wild yam *(Diascorea),* which is rich in natural molecules that can be chemically changed into a variety of steroid hormones, including DHEA, testosterone, progesterone, and the three human estrogens.

You can't get a significant amount of these hormones from eating Mexican yams or using creams based on them directly, though. The human body does not possess the chemical cofactors required to convert them to useful hormones. These can only be found in a properly equipped labaratory.

This important scientific fact has not stopped a few entrepreneurs from marketing yam products as sources of various steroid hormones. Please don't be fooled! If you purchase a progesterone or DHEA cream, make sure it actually contains these substances and not just unprocessed Mexican yam.

Dioscorea is another plant remedy used in traditional medicine for hundreds, perhaps thousands of years. Some of these uses have been in disorders of the menstrual cycle. Many women have told me that dioscorea has helped them feel better. These improvements, while real, do not appear to be due to any content of DHEA, progesterone, testosterone, or estrogens. If these hormones are present, they must have been added to the dioscorea preparation.

of molecular structure than horse or other animal estrogens. Even the strongest phytoestrogens have at most 1 to 2% the potency of human estrogens.

For these reasons, phytoestrogens can't really replace human hormones. It's also very unlikely they will have the same degree of beneficial effect on bone, heart and blood vessels, and brain. Phytoestrogens are similar to natural estrogens in one way, though. Because they, too, are unpatentable, phytoestrogens simply haven't undergone the extensive research that patentable "hormones" have.

This most definitely does *not* mean that herbal menopause remedies containing phytoestrogens are useless. A very long tradition of human use tells even the most skeptical research scientist that there's probably something there. This is proving to be the case with several items available at natural food stores, such as:

- **Chaste Berry** *(Vitex agnus)*. Chaste berry appears to act in areas of the brain that regulate pituitary hormones, *increasing secretion of LH* and *decreasing FSH* (see Chapter 2). This results in a relative increase in progesterone and a relative decrease in estrogens. Chaste berry can be particularly useful for PMS (premenstrual syndrome) and heavy menstrual periods, as well as symptoms of the perimenopause.

- **Black Cohosh** *(Cimicifuga racemosa),* a phytoestrogen-containing plant, has a long history of use by Native Americans to relieve menstrual cramps. European botanical experts find it particularly useful against depression at the time of menopause. Phytochemicals in black cohosh both *decrease LH* (thereby shifting the estrogen/progesterone ratio towards estrogens, an effect opposite in some ways to chaste berry) and *occupy estradiol receptors.*

- **Dong Quai** *(Angelica sinensis),* an ancient Asian herbal remedy, appears to act as an *estrogen modulator* through the ability of its phytoestrogens to occupy estrogen receptor sites. If estrogen levels are low, *angelica's* phytoestrogens, although much weaker than estrogen, provide some estrogen stimulus by filling unoccupied receptor sites; if estrogen levels are too high, these same phytoestrogens block some of the estrogen by occupying the same receptor sites.

- **Licorice** *(Glycyrrhiza glabra)* appears to modulate estrogen action in the same way as dong quai.
- **Panax Ginseng** has been shown to have estrogenic effects on the vaginal lining, helping to relieve dryness and pain. Ginseng has been traditionally used in Asia for a wide variety of menstrual cycle disorders, as well as an anti-aging botanical.

It's very likely that many more herbs that influence menstrual cycle hormones will appear in pharmacies and natural food stores over the next few years. However, as you've read above, the principal effects (and traditional uses) of these phytoestrogen-containing herbs appear to be on disorders of menstruation and symptoms of the menopause and perimenopause. With the exception of ginseng, there's not much emphasis on long-term use after the menopause, which is the point of both patentable "HRT" and the more body-friendly NHR. In my experience, phytoestrogens and NHR overlap, but don't duplicate each other. Each has its own valuable place in natural health care.

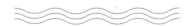

RESOURCES

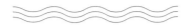

How to Obtain Natural Hormones

BECAUSE THEY ARE NOT manufactured by multinational pharmaceutical companies and endorsed with FDA's incredibly costly stamp of "approval" ($450 million or more for a single "approval," according to a recent Government Accounting Office report), natural hormones do not normally appear on the shelves of most pharmacies. But they're not impossible, illegal, or even difficult to get. You just have to know who to ask and what to ask for.

Some natural hormones (progesterone, DHEA, melatonin) are available over the counter in pharmacies and natural food stores. Others (estrone, estradiol, estriol) are available only on prescription by medical doctors (MDs), osteopathic doctors (DOs), and in some states, naturopathic doctors (NDs). One (testosterone) is only available on prescription as a "controlled substance." There's very little logic behind it all, but as the saying goes, "that's government work."

Compounding Pharmacists: Back to the Future

Natural hormones that are not available in over-the-counter preparations can be obtained on prescription from one of the growing number of *compounding pharmacies* in the United States. Compounding pharmacists prepare the hormones for each patient according to their doctor's prescription in the form (pills, capsules, creams, gels, pellets, and implants) best suited to the patient's individual needs.

In the centuries before the pharmaceutical industry took over the manufacturing of nearly all drugs, all pharmacists were compounding pharmacists. As recently as the early 1940s, most drugs and natural compounds were prepared this way. But by the 1980s, most pharmacists had been relegated to the role of pill counters.

As everyone knows, the current system basically works like this: the doctor writes a prescription for a standardized commercial drug like Premarin, and either calls the pharmacist or gives it to the patient who then hands it to the pharm-acist at the local drug store. The pharmacist, who keeps a supply of Premarin on hand, reads the prescription, opens a bottle of Premarin pills of the pre-scribed strength (usually 0.625 mg or 1.25 mg), counts out the pre-scribed number of pills, puts them in a bottle with the patient's name and dosing instructions on it, and hands the bottle to the patient. In many cases a vending machine could do the job just as well.

Fortunately, compounding pharmacies have been undergoing a rebirth, caused by rapidly growing public demand for more nat-ural and more individualized health care, and by economic neces-sity for the traditional, small personal-service pharmacy. Consumers are increasingly dissatisfied with "nothing but drugs," and are seeking out natural remedies in ever-increasing numbers.

Compounding pharmacies are literally the only sources for pre-scription natural hormones and other prescription natural items. But even drug-prescribing doctors are increasingly frustrated with the limited selection of "approved" drug preparations, and are working with compounding pharmacists in increasing numbers to develop unique preparations and "delivery systems."

Many small, traditional, personal-service pharmacies were liter-ally being driven out of business by cost-cutting insurance com-panies, "managed care" organizations, and HMOs that sign contracts with giant drugstore chains to provide massive quanti-ties of deeply discounted drugs, or even opening their own mail-in drug outlets. With rapidly increasing consumer demand, the path to economic survival for smaller personal-service pharmacies became obvious: a return to traditional pharmaceutical com-pounding.

Today's compounding pharmacists can produce literally what-ever the doctor orders, usually in a variety of forms that best suit the patient's needs. Need some "triple estrogen" in capsules? Testosterone in a gel? You simply have your doctor write a prescription, which you present to a compounding pharmacist.

Compounding pharmacists have access to bulk quantities of high-quality natural hormones (and other substances) as well as the equipment to process them. They measure out appropriate doses and put them into whichever medium the doctor prescribes.

The pills, capsules, creams, etc, produced by a compounding pharmacist are virtually indistinguishable from the mass-produced variety, except that they usually don't come with the chemical colorings and shapes the pharmaceutical industry uses to distinguish its products from the competition and discourage "counterfeiting." As an added "bonus," a compounding pharmacist can leave out all unnecessary chemical flavors and preservatives, as well as coloring chemicals, and can individualize "bases" according to a patient's allergies and sensitivities.

The quality of individually prepared natural hormones or drugs produced by a compounding pharmacist is excellent for several reasons:.

- Compounding pharmacists are often more extensively educated than pharmacists who are just "pill-counters." They've taken special training in modern compounding methods.
- They have that extra motivation borne of having to satisfy each individual customer for their individualized prescription. A primary motivation for many non-compounding pharmacists is keeping a "third-party payer" happy. "Happiness" for third-party payers means always the lowest price possible, with "patient satisfaction" a very secondary consideration.
- Every compounding pharmacy is licensed and inspected by its State Pharmacy Board, just like all other pharmacies.
- Materials used by compounding pharmacies are the same quality used by the major pharmaceutical companies. All materials used are subject to FDA inspection and the agency's Good Manufacturing Procedures code.

It's no surprise that FDA and the pharmaceutical industry would like to see competition from compounding pharmacists eliminated, and have made significant efforts to squash this valuable health resource. So far, this repression has been stalled in Congress, thanks to the vigorous lobbying efforts of representatives of the compounding pharmacists, knowledgeable medical professionals and consumers, and others concerned with preserving one of the last outposts of health care freedom in the USA.

How to Locate a Compounding Pharmacist

There are compounding pharmacies all over the country, and locating one nearby is not difficult. If there is no compounding pharmacy nearby, nearly all transactions can be carried out via mail, phone and/or fax.

The easiest way to locate a compounding pharmacist is to contact the International Academy of Compounding Pharmacists (IACP) or the Professional Compounding Centers of America, Inc. (PCCA).

PCCA provides compounding pharmacists with support in the form of training, equipment, chemicals, and technical consultation on difficult compounding problems. At present, more than 1,900 compounding pharmacists in the US, Canada, Australia, and New Zealand are members of PCCA. For information about PCCA, including a listing of compounding pharmacists:

Telephone: 800-331-2498 **Fax:** 800-874-5760
Internet: www.compassnet.com/~pcca/

The IACP can be contacted at:
Telephone: 800-927-4227 **Fax:** 281-495-0602
Postal Address: PO Box 1365
Sugar Land, TX 77487
Internet: www.compassnet.com/~iacp/

How to Get a Medical Doctor to Prescribe Natural Hormones

The quickest and most efficient way is to visit a medical doctor or osteopath who is a member of the American College for Advancement in Medicine (ACAM). All members of this professional organization are skilled and knowledgeable in the prescription and use of natural hormones. ACAM members have studied and listened to discussions by dozens of experts (even including myself on occasion) concerning the biochemistry, effects, and uses of natural hormones. For a referral to an ACAM doctor near you, contact ACAM at:

Telephone: 1-800-532-3688
Address: 23121 Verdugo Drive/Suite 204
Laguna Hills, CA 92653
Internet: www.acam.org

Because most of their hormone- and drug-related information comes from pharmaceutical sales reps, medical journals supported by pharmaceutical company advertising, or pharmaceutical company sponsored conventions, the average "conventional" medical doctor in the United States knows virtually nothing about using natural hormones. To many of these doctors, natural hormones sound like the latest natural food fad: "Estrogen and progesterone made from yam steroids! Give me a break! Let's see those placebo-controlled, double-blind studies. Let's see that FDA 'approval.' Let's see those free samples!" All too often, "conventional" medical doctors are intimidated by their state medical boards, medical societies, or other peer groups, all of whom still disapprove of "natural remedies."

Fortunately, like the rest of us, increasing numbers of medical doctors are seeing through the smoke and mirrors offered up by the government/pharmaceutical complex. Many of these doctors have taken it upon themselves to learn about natural hormones and to recommend them to their patients in preference to pharmaceutical "hormones."

Many other medical doctors, though perhaps less knowledgeable about natural hormones, are dissatisfied with the "approved" methods of treating menopause, because these so often prove to be unpleasant and possibly dangerous. These doctors are open-minded enough to recognize that the pharmaceutical industry does not have all the answers. If asked to prescribe natural hormones and provided with supporting documentation and dosing options, they're often happy to oblige, because they're always looking for better ways to help their patients.

If your doctor is interested but hesitant to prescribe natural hormones, put him or her in touch with a compounding pharmacist, who can both reassure and provide education. Having such a consultation with a knowledgeable professional, who can explain the advantages of natural hormones and provide some dosing guidelines is usually enough to convince most skeptical doctors to at least give natural hormones a try.

Other Medical Alternatives

Although the American Medical Association would probably like you to believe otherwise, there are qualified medical professionals who have letters other than MD after their name. Many of these doctors, known as naturopaths and osteopaths, have a far better understanding of natural hormones, and usually considerably more experience in using them than the average "regular" MD.

Naturopathic Physicians. Naturopathic medicine is based on the belief and observation that the human body possesses enormous power to heal itself when given the correct natural materials and energies. Natural hormones are certainly among these materials.

After earning an undergraduate degree (BA or BS) including pre-medical requirements, such as chemistry, biochemistry, biology, and physics, naturopathic physicians go on to a 4-year graduate level, accredited naturopathic school of medicine, where they earn an ND degree upon graduation. NDs are educated in all the same sciences as MDs, although with less emphasis on drugs, radiation, and surgery, but much more emphasis on nutrition, botanical remedies, manipulation, homeopathy, acupuncture, psychology, and other holistic and nontoxic therapies. Naturopathic physicians place strong emphasis on disease prevention, lifestyle change, and optimizing wellness.

Before licensure, naturopathic physicians must complete at least 4,000 hours of study in specified subject areas and then pass a series of rigorous professional board exams. Although naturopathic physicians can be found in every US state and Canadian province, they're currently licensed by state boards only in Alaska, Arizona, Connecticut, Hawaii, Maine, Montana, New Hampshire, Oregon, Utah, Vermont, Washington, and the District of Columbia. In Canada, naturopaths are licensed in British Columbia,

Manitoba, Ontario, and Saskatchewan.

To locate a naturopathic physician, contact the American Association of Naturopathic Physicians (AANP) at:

Telephone: 206-328-8510
Address: 2366 Eastlake Ave/Suite 322
Seattle, WA 98102
Internet: www.infinite.org/Naturopathic.Physician/

Osteopathic Physicians. After earning an undergraduate degree (BA or BS), doctors of osteopathic medicine graduate from a 4-year osteopathic medical school with a DO degree. Their training and accreditation is similar to that which medical doctors receive. Most osteopaths are primary care physicians, but many specialize in such areas as internal medicine, surgery, pediatrics, radiology, or pathology. Residencies in these areas typically require an additional 2 to 6 years of training beyond medical school.

DOs differ from MDs primarily in their emphasis on a "whole person" and preventive approach to the practice of medicine. Rather than treat specific symptoms, as many conventional "allopathic" MDs usually do, a DO is trained to focus on the body's various systems—particularly the musculoskeletal system—and how they interact with each other. Although DOs can and do prescribe conventional drugs, they are more likely to be open to and knowledgeable about natural remedies, including natural hormone replacement.

Osteopaths are licensed in all US states and Canadian provinces to practice medicine and prescribe drugs. To find an osteopath, a good starting point is the American Osteopathic Association (AOA) or the Canadian Osteopathic Association (COA):

American Osteopathic Association
Address: 142 E. Ontario Street
Chicago, IL 60611-2864
Telephone: 312-380-5800
Internet: www.am-osteo-assn.org

Canadian Osteopathic Association
Address: 575 Waterloo Street
London, Ontario N6B2R2
Telephone: 519-439-5521

Laboratory Testing. Many laboratories test hormones in blood, and a few check levels in saliva. I prefer to use the *24-hour urine test,* because nearly all hormones are secreted in "bursts" and "pulses," and a single "blood draw" or saliva collection (or even two or three of them) may not provide a representative sample.

The lab I work with uses the most up-to-date equipment (including mass spectroscopy, for the technically inclined) and offers multiple steroid hormone panels at exceptionally good prices. This laboratory is:

Meridian Valley Clinical Laboratories
Address: 515 West Harrison
Kent, Washington 98032
Telephones: 800-234-6825 or 206-859-8700
Fax: 206-859-1135

A F T E R W O R D

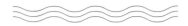

I HOPE THIS BOOK HAS BEEN HELPFUL. If you've read this far, I suspect you'll never use any hormone replacement except the natural kind. Hopefully, those pregnant mares can be turned out to pasture!

As you've read, many women I work with have already applied the under-lying principles of natural hormone replacement to all other aspects of their personal health care:

- They've eliminated (or minimized) the use of drugs.
- They've learned how to work with vitamins, minerals, and botanical remedies.
- They've learned to harness the natural energies contained in homeopathic remedies.
- They're working with their own natural energies through acupuncture, massage, chiropractic, and osteopathy.

Natural hormone replacement is only a part of an overall natural health care picture. Certainly, drugs and surgery have their place in health care (usually in emergencies or for short-term situations), but our bodies are natural, and do best over the long run with natural materials and energies. We don't get headaches because of an aspirin deficiency, and nervousness doesn't happen because our bodies need Valium.

The quality of our food and water is also very important:

- Whole, natural foods, processed as little as possible, with no chemical flavorings, colorings, or preservatives (again, molecules our bodies aren't designed to handle) are always best for the best of health.
- Eliminating refined sugar and artificial (chemical) sweeteners

is important, too.

- Although coffee and tobacco are natural, they're laden with chemicals. Coffee is the world's most herbicide- and pesticide-sprayed crop, and cigarettes have been disclosed to have more than 400 chemical additives.
- The water we drink should be free of *all* added chemicals, including chlorine and fluoride. Beer and wine in moderation don't seem to be a problem, but any more than a little *distilled* alcohol is.

Of course, it's a cliché that "just because it's natural doesn't mean it's safe." We can drown in clean, pure water. But over the course of tens of thousands of human generations, our ancestors have learned and passed down the knowledge of which mushroom or herb will poison us and which will help heal. And no one can argue that natural therapies are not incredibly safer than drugs.

So, if you haven't done so already, please explore the many other aspects of natural health care, especially natural self-care for yourself and your family. With natural self-care, you'll likely find illness to be a much less frequent visitor, and you'll feel more alive and energetic, ready to face the rest of life and whatever tasks you have yet to accomplish here on Earth.

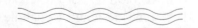

I N D E X

NATURAL HORMONE REPLACEMENT/INDEX

A P P E N D I X

ALTHOUGH WE HAVE QUOTED an estrone-estriol ratio ranging from 10%-10%-80% to 20%-20%-60% throughout this book, recent preliminary work with a small number of women well before menopausal age has show that, if anything, the early-1980s estimate of estriol's predominance may have been too conservative! As shown in this graph, researchers at Meridian Valley Laboratories* have recently demonstrated that tha actual ratio of the three estrogens on days 10 to 12 of the menstrual cycle (when estrone and estradiol are at or near their peak levels) in these women is closer to 3%-7%-90%. This research is now being extended to a much larger group of women to further explore this important question.

---

* Schliesman BD, Robinson LM. Serum estrogens: quantitative analysis of the concentration of estriol compared to estradiol and estrone. Meridian Valley Laboratory, Kent, WA. Data on file.

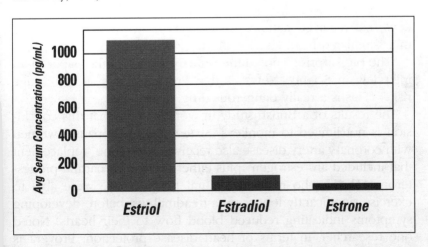

Relative Amounts of Estrogens in Normal Premenopausal Women

Provera and Heart Disease:
"Worse Than No Treatment at All"

Heart disease is responsible for at least three-fourths of the deaths in postmenopausal women. Although much evidence suggests that estrogen replacement helps reduce the risks associated with heart disease, new data confirms that the common practice of taking the synthetic progestin Provera along with "estrogen" to minimize the risk of endometrial cancer may be increasing women's risk of suffering a heart attack to an unacceptable level. Natural progesterone, however, provides cancer protection but carries no such risk.

This conclusion comes from a new study carried out in rhesus monkeys at the Oregon Regional Primate Research Center. Eighteen monkeys had their ovaries removed to simulate menopause. They were then put on a hormone replacement regimen that included estradiol plus either Provera or natural progesterone. After 4 weeks, the researchers injected a substance that causes coronary arteries (which supply the heart with blood) to constrict, cutting off the flow of blood to the heart muscle.

The researchers reported that the animals receiving Provera would have died within minutes had they not received a protective drug treatment. The same thing happened in those animals that received no hormone replacement. By contrast, those monkeys that received natural progesterone quickly recovered from their simulated heart attack with no protective drug treatment.

"The big surprise," noted the primary author of the paper in an interview in Science News, is that Provera poses such a "huge risk." "This is a really dangerous drug."

The results of a British study in women show that this conclusion is not limited to monkeys. Sixteen postmenopausal women with coronary artery disease also received "hormone" replacement that included an "estrogen" plus either Provera or natural progesterone. Those who received natural progesterone were able to exercise significantly longer on a treadmill test before developing symptoms indicating reduced blood flow to their hearts. Noted one researcher, in terms of heart disease protection, Provera is "worse than no treatment at all."